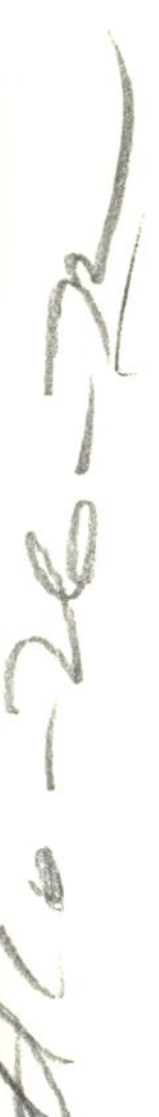

Essay Index

FRONTIERS IN MEDICINE

The March of Medicine, 1950

NUMBER XV OF
THE NEW YORK ACADEMY OF MEDICINE
LECTURES TO THE LAITY

FRONTIERS IN MEDICINE

The March of Medicine, 1950

The New York Academy of Medicine

Essay Index Reprint Series

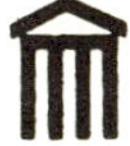

BOOKS FOR LIBRARIES PRESS
FREEPORT, NEW YORK

The Committee on Lectures to the Laity is composed of Harold B. Keyes, M.D., Chairman, Norton S. Brown, M.D., and E. Everett Bunzel, M.D., representing the Committee on Medical Information; Leo Mayer, M.D., Lawrence S. Kubie, M.D., and Rustin McIntosh, M.D., representing the Committee on Medical Education; Frederick R. Bailey, M.D., representing the Committee on Public Health Relations; I. H. Goldberger, M.D., representing the Board of Education of New York City. Iago Galdston, M.D., is Executive Secretary.

INTERNATIONAL STANDARD BOOK NUMBER:

0-8369-2113-5

LIBRARY OF CONGRESS CATALOG CARD NUMBER:

70-142675

PRINTED IN THE UNITED STATES OF AMERICA

FOREWORD

"All other knowledge is hurtful to him who has not the science of honesty and good nature."
—Montaigne

IN THIS SPIRIT, the Committee on Medical Information launched the fifteenth series of Laity Lectures. The enthusiastic attendance justified the hopes of the Committee, and the high quality of the speeches. The subject matter proved timely and was an intellectual stimulus to all present. The lay and professional guests of honor showed continued interest and pleasure in these enjoyable dinners and conferences.

"Frontiers in Psychiatry" was an intriguing subject for the first lecture, and held undivided attention, and alerted us to keep abreast of the speaker's subject. Dr. Franz Alexander was as stimulating as his subject. "Whatever that be which thinks, understands, wills and acts, it is something celestial and divine" (Cicero).

Dr. David Seegal encouraged both old and young with his talk Methuselah: Myth or Promise! "No wise man ever wished to be younger" (Swift).

The Anniversary Discourse of The New York Academy of Medicine was delivered by Dr. Laurence H. Snyder whose theme was "Frontiers in Genetics."

"Machines That Work Like Men" was an exciting discourse by Dr. John H. Gibbons, Jr. One wonders to what length machines will, in the future, either stimulate or stultify our minds. "The wise are instructed by reason" (Cicero).

Dr. Selman A. Waksman again alerted us to the most

recent work on the amazing antibiotics, and opened new fields of thought on health preservation and the curative process in disease. "The disease and its medicine are like two factions in a besieged Town" (Jeffrey).

The George R. Siedenburg Memorial Lecture, given by Dr. Thomas M. Rivers, of Rockefeller Institute for Medical Research, was a report on the basic methods of medical research. Speaking at The New York Academy of Medicine, during a Laity Lecture series, Dr. Conant, of Harvard, reiterated the need for research in basic and pure science, and urged all to support such work without restraint, and regardless of immediate return.

We were especially fortunate in the men who presided at these lectures; Dr. Robert P. Knight, Dr. Frank G. Boudreau, Dr. Harry L. Shapiro, Dr. Herbert B. Wilcox, Jr., Dr. René J. Dubos, and Dr. Alan Gregg.

The subject matter of the lectures was so stimulating that the questions from the audiences proved to be in greater number than could be answered in the allotted time.

We are grateful to our speakers, our chairmen, and to the various committees who arranged the programs.

It has been a privilege to be present at these lectures and meet the distinguished scientists and guests, who participated.

HAROLD BROWN KEYES, M.D.

New York
September, 1951

INTRODUCTION

THE TITLE of this volume, *Frontiers in Medicine,* is descriptive of its content, and is in a sense inspired. Here six distinguished contributors, each at the forefront of his specialty, describes in particular terms the "ground that has been gained, held, and consolidated" therein in recent years. Each essay is in itself a comprehensive recitation. Collectively, however, they convey a something greater than that sum of their respective tales. They mirror the pattern of progress in medicine. This pattern is not consistent with what it is ordinarily thought to be. Nor does it quite conform to the picture of medical progress depicted in the histories of medicine.

The realities of experience differ from the descriptions given of them in later times. In these essays experience is verbalized as it emerges and the result is no less fascinating than instructive. Thus, experience—some would term it progress—is apparently not consistent. It moves, like the wind, where it listeth. And its results are in a large measure unpredictable. The moral of this, in these days of universal planning is not without significance!

In the first of the essays, presented by Dr. Alexander, we observe that the specialty originally restricted to the care and study of the severely disturbed patient has now extended its scope of application and concern to include the study and the manipulation of the so-called normal. This extension is referred to as the "sociological implications of modern psychiatry." We are now familiar with the expressions "psychological warfare," and "group dynamics," both of which are instances of sociological psychology. Dr. Alexander most ably dilates on this subject. Here we need only underscore the fact that "progress" in psychiatry has not merely followed the path of better care of the mentally and emotionally sick patient, but has in truly unexpected ways led off into seemingly remote terrains.

Recently the Academy sponsored a conference of Panic and Morale, where, in most urgent and telling ways the data of the social sciences and of psychiatry were pooled by the disciples of both disciplines, in an attempt to lay bare the sources of that most contagious of all disorders of the mind and spirit to which man is subject. Also, and because it is implied in the quest, the conference sought to define morale, which appears to be the very antidote to panic, and a positive good in itself.

The point here to be underscored is the ultimate deviation of a discipline which, initiated in the care of the unfortunate lunatic, has now become a science potential of great social good and evil. Psychiatry can be applied both as an offensive and as a defensive weapon in war. It can also be utilized in the upbuilding of morale in the absence of war, and may even thus serve to dissipate the fears, anxieties, and aggressions that contribute to the engenderment of war.

The contribution of Dr. David Seegal, "Methuselah: Myth or Promise," illustrates as effectively the thesis here advanced that medicine progresses in unpredictable and unanticipated ways. Geriatrics is a "specialty" of recent origin. It is a *by-product* rather than the direct result of medical progress. Our population is now weighted with a high percentage of persons in the later stages of life. Phrasing it crudely, this relative preponderance of older persons is due to the circumstance that fewer in our community are permitted to die in early adulthood. Seemingly this should be all to the good. To the good it is, but not all. For among those surviving there are many who are sick and ailing. We are therefore faced with *new* problems, how, as an instance, we can gain longevity free of degeneration and illness, and also how, in the interim, we can best deal with the older sick individual.

It would not do to make this introduction too long, and there is really no need to belabor the point here made. Given the tangent the reader can follow it with ease in the essays published in this volume. He will find its tracings in each contribution. It really could not be otherwise, for it is ingrained in the emergence, not only of medicine but of every science and discipline. I am sure the Curies did not anticipate the A-bomb. Nor did Professor Waksman (when he began to study soil as a living economy) foresee the "cures" now effected by the antibiotics he helped to produce. Dr. Thomas Rivers, by the very nature of the subject matter of his lecture, "Concepts and Methods of Medical Research," most directly expounds the thesis underscored in this introduction.

One final word and that in the nature of an apology. Why the emphasis on the unpredictability of medical progress? Immediately, because it might serve to restrain the enthusiasm of those who would "plan for progress" on a long range; but more pertinently, because in this emphasis lies the rationale of the Academy's Lectures to the Laity. Knowledge alone does not suffice. Indeed it may prove an encumbrance. What is needed, in addition, is understanding. Understanding not infrequently points to conclusions which contradict and deny the patent "meaning" of the known fact.

It has been the consistent aim of the Academy to advance understanding *in* the spread of knowledge. In these respects this volume of essays is an outstanding instance of an aim well achieved.

We need not be too restrained in our praise, for the credit is due entirely to the contributors, who have come from "far and wide" and have given freely and generously of their knowledge and experience. To them, and also to the membership of the Committee which organizes these lectures, we are deeply indebted.

IAGO GALDSTON, M.D.

New York
September, 1951

CONTENTS

FRONTIERS IN MEDICINE

FRONTIERS IN PSYCHIATRY

By Franz Alexander, M.D.

PSYCHIATRY, not long ago the stepchild of medicine, has become in the last two decades one of the focal points of significant advance in medical science. This progress is taking place on two borderline fields: between psychiatry and the other medical sciences; and between psychiatry and the social sciences.

Originally, psychiatry was restricted to the care and study of the psychotic, the severely disturbed patient whose personality functions have deteriorated to a degree that he requires custodial care. His thought processes and feelings are so different from those of healthy persons that common sense cannot grasp them. Only after psychiatrists, under the leadership of Freud, turned their attention to the much larger group of neurotics whose deviation is circumscribed to certain areas but who otherwise in their feeling, thinking, and behavior closely resemble average persons, did the science of human motivations—psychodynamics—begin to develop. Psychodynamics explains human behavior in the terms of psychological cause and effect. It attempts to formulate the basic principles which govern mental processes in the same way that physics formulates the laws which govern the behavior of inanimate bodies. In precision, psychodynamics is of course still far behind such sciences as hydrodynamics or electrodynamics.

Psychodynamics found its application in three fields: in explaining individual behavior and treating its disturbances such as psychoses and neuroses; in the study of the influence of emotions upon bodily processes and organic diseases; and, finally, in the exploration of group phenomena. The first field is that of psychiatry and psychology; the second is called psychosomatic medicine; and the third is that of the social sciences. I had the opportunity to discuss the first two topics a few years ago in The New York Academy of Medicine and shall limit myself now to the sociological implications of modern psychiatry.

As a theory of human personality, psychoanalysis has a bearing not only upon medicine but also upon education and the social sciences. Man is a member of society and his social behavior can be understood only in terms of his own nature. At the same time personality to a large degree is a product of social influences. Everyone is born with a basic biological equipment, but, from birth on, the environment, at first through parental influences, later through more extended channels, has a permanent molding influence upon this inherited substratum and profoundly determines the development of the personality. In this field, also, Freud was a pioneer and made fundamental discoveries. Though many anthropologists knew and described in great detail the two basic taboos in primitive societies—not to have sexual relations with a woman belonging to the same totem group and not to kill the totem animal which is the symbol of the father—Freud was the first to explain their meaning. He recognized that these two basic laws are defenses against what he called the Oedipus complex. Every social organization must defend itself against these primitive tendencies. The unity of the family can be preserved only if the sexual interest of the sons becomes diverted from the female members of the family, because only thus can the rivalry between father and sons be circumvented. In this way, the integrity of the family is saved, and a social group is created through exogamous marriage. The family is the cell of the society. Families become united through exogamy into clans, then into tribes, and finally into nations. Freud showed how the emotional structure of the human personality was influenced by social institutions.

Freud tried to apply psychoanalytic knowledge to the understanding of social organization. He distinguished two basic dynamic factors in social life: the dependence of the members of an organized group upon their leader, and their identification with each other and the leader.

The leadership principle seems to be as fundamental to society as it is to biological organisms, in which it manifests itself in the differentiation of the head end and the tail end of the body. The nature of leadership may show extreme variations, but in every society there is some kind of leadership, such as monarchy, rule by the elite—aristocracy, or democratic government. It is not difficult to recognize the utility of leadership; it is needed for the coordination of the activities of the group members. Utility and reason, however, usually exert their influence secondarily. It is not likely that one fine day people discovered by logical deduction the usefulness of leadership. Leadership evolves spontaneously in every social organization and must have much more primitive sources than deductive logic. Freud has pointed out that the emotional dependence of the members upon the leader is a derivative of the child's dependence upon the father. The emotional nature of this dependence can best be observed in dangerous emergency situations. In danger, human beings have the tendency to regress to an earlier phase of development, to seek security by turning for help to a leader as they turned toward the adults in their childhood. In times of external danger, people are inclined to turn for help to a strong government and to renounce, at least temporarily, some of their freedoms and privileges. This phenomenon can best be observed in democracies; it is not so obvious in societies where the central government regulates the lives of people all the time.

Emotional need for dependence is, however, not the only factor which makes peoples accept leadership. They do this also for utilitarian reasons. In emergency, when quick action is needed, execution of decisions made on the basis of reliable information is imperative. This calls for a central executive. Leadership probably evolves both from utility and from emotional needs. As soon as the danger relaxes, people accustomed to a greater amount of self-government usually begin to resent centralized leadership and clamor again for their previous state of greater independence. Dependence explains, however, only the need of being led and not leadership itself. The psychology of the leader, the wish to lead, also has deep emotional sources and can be retraced to the parental propensities of man. Maternal instinct is not the only manifestation of this biologically rooted propensity. The father's care for the family, either by providing food or by defending it from attack, is just as basic. Both maternal instinct and paternal care for the family are manifestations of the general biological tendency of the mature organism (which can no longer add anything to its own growth) to expend excess energy for the sake of others, primarily for its own progeny. Every social organization is based on these two fundamental biological tendencies of the organism: childish dependence and the parental instinct to take care of the progeny.

All this becomes clear if one realizes that social organization is one of the means by which life is preserved. Darwin considered man's social propensities as one of his greatest advantages in the struggle for survival. The value of social cooperation is known also to insects, which give man serious competition for the possession of the earth. Survival requires different types of activities, such as fighting enemies, building shelter against the rigors of nature, producing food, and the preparation of tools. The value of specialization of function is obvious. A specialist performs his assignments with greater precision and speed than a Jack-of-all-trades. Specialized functions must of course be coordinated with each other in a sensible way suitable for serving the needs of society. Some form of government is therefore indispensable in organized society, particularly when, with a high degree of specialization, the division of labor becomes so advanced that the members of the group become less self-sufficient and more dependent upon each other for survival.

Just like leadership, this interdependence of the members of the group has its rational basis and is the inevitable result of the specialization of social functions. Like leadership, it has a primitive origin, which Freud described as the identification of the members with each other and with their leader. Clan and tribal spirit and nationalism are well-known examples of this emotional cement of society. By belonging to the same group under a common leader or leadership the members are akin to each other. Each can place himself in the other member's position; what helps the members is to his advantage—what threatens the others endangers him, too.

In a highly specialized society, mutual interdependence is greater than in a primitive society and yet it is less transparent. To recognize the common interests requires detached intellectual insight. As soon as groups become distinct from one another because of divergent social functions and status, the differences make the identification more difficult and obscure the basic fact that for the sake of their own welfare they have to consider the interests of others.

Nothing proves this better than the eternal struggle between groups and classes belonging to the same nation. Both parties are inclined to overlook their common interests and each tries to improve its own position without consideration for the other. Mediation is seldom successful. The stark fact that the employer can profit only by considering the welfare of the employee and the employee can maintain his own welfare only by considering the interests of the employer is not understood with sufficient clarity by either group. It is true, of course, that in complex modern society, the precise evaluation of common and divergent interests is not a simple task. The natural inclination of each group is first to seek its own advantage and at best to give only secondary consideration to the other group. To recognize the fact that, by compromising to some extent, one's own interest may ultimately be benefited even from the selfish point of view, is not supported by any spontaneous emotion. This insight can only be achieved by detached logical operation. Furthermore, there is no way of gauging precisely how far one should go in abandoning one's own immediate advantage. There is no question that exploitation of the weaker group by the more powerful is a common and permanent evil of social life. In certain periods and in certain societies these discrepancies become so great that the more basic parallelism of interests is completely overlooked. The theory that class struggle is the essence of social life is an outgrowth of a one-sided evaluation of social interaction in modern society.

Both Marx and Pareto were impressed by the same fact, although they came to entirely opposite conclusions. The Utopian solution of Marx was to terminate class struggle in two steps: the first, to establish the iron dictatorship of one class, the proletariat. This would lead eventually to the second step—a classless society. He never recognized the basic contradiction in his view. If class struggle is the essence of social life, it must be based upon human psychology—upon the fact that people selfishly pursue their own interests. Why should the dictatorship of one of the groups lead to a millennium of social justice? Obviously it can be achieved only by a miraculous change of human nature.

Pareto views history as the repetition of the same cycle. Political power is always exercised by a forceful elite which imposes upon the rest of society its domination under the guise of a deceptive ideology that makes the suppressed classes believe the leaders are their protectors. The rulers gradually take their own rationalizations seriously, they become weak and decadent and gradually yield to the pressure of hungry power-seeking up-starts who replace them and dominate society by a new set of deceptions. Pareto never considers that constructive type of leadership, which is the sublimation or extension of the parental instinct to take care of others.

Pareto however, is more consistent than Marx. Both depart from the same fundamental thesis that society is ruled by selfish interest and force. Marx, in contradiction to his own thesis, seeks the termination of the external cycle of class struggle by a magic formula, introducing social justice without considering a change in human attitudes. If it is true that the only dominant force in social life is violence and subjugation of the weak, Pareto's theory is more consistent than that of Marx, but neither of them considers those cohesive emotional forces in social life which Freud described: the dependence on the leader and the primitive identification of the members with each other. Moreover, neither Pareto nor Marx recognized sufficiently the interaction of these emotional factors with the utilitarian bases of social organization. Pareto accepts the rule of the strong;

he sees social injustice as an essential feature of every society. Marx, in his Utopian plan, aims for a society based on social justice, yet in his fundamental assumptions, so far as past history is concerned, he does not give any place to a sense of justice in social life. Sense of justice appears as a *deus ex machina* from the moment that the rule of the labor class begins.

It is of great interest to explore the psychological background of these distortions in social theory. This will necessitate the examination of the emotional sources of the sense of justice.

Its roots go back to the early experiences of the child in the family, which is, in a sense, the most primitive form of society. The sibling's welfare depends upon parental love and care. Because of the dependent nature of the child, he watches his own prerogatives keenly and considers all brothers and sisters as competitors. Through identification with them, and also by more complex psychodynamic processes, the original sibling rivalry will be overlaid by loyalty and often by a protective attitude assumed by older toward younger siblings. Behind these surface attitudes, the original rivalries remain latent and become manifest whenever one child receives obvious parental preference.

A readiness to compromise and to renounce unlimited self-seeking can only be achieved when the parents assume an undiscriminatory and just attitude toward all the children. Age differences, of course, prevent each child's being treated in exactly the same way. The youngest child has certain privileges resulting from his greater dependence; the older ones receive privileges so far as freedom is concerned. The judicious distribution of parental favors and filial duties is obviously the basis of the sense of justice which later becomes important in social life. It is the only efficient defense against mutual envy: that of the siblings for each other and later between competing social groups. Equality before the law is the social equivalent of the impartiality of the parents. Whenever the socioeconomic mechanism, which never functions with ideal precision, gets out of gear, the original sibling rivalries are reactivated and social groups revolt and attack each other. They vindicate their destructive and aggressive actions on the grounds that social justice has been violated.

I am fully aware how difficult it is in these days of wars, social crises, and atomic weapons, to put faith in the constructive possibilities of human nature. Today, the situation is diametrically opposite to the one which prevailed at the turn of the century when Freud called attention to the asocial nucleus of the human personality. He advanced his theory when the Western world enjoyed a period of relative peace and material well-being, when people complacently considered themselves civilized and spoke contemptuously of the barbarism of the past and the savages of primitive cultures. Freud was considered a degrader of human nature. His opinion, however, concerning the power of man's unconscious impulses has been vindicated on a large historical scale sooner than he expected.

Two world wars with ensuing deterioration of social standards, the return in Central and Eastern Europe to the most barbaric phases of human history, the revival of the most primitive forms of tyranny and minority rule, and, above all, the general preoccupation with weapons of destruction—all these demonstrate only too clearly that, behind his civilized veneer, man harbors in himself an asocial nucleus more destructive than the atomic nucleus which he has recently put into the service of his own destructive purposes. Today, few would question man's asocial qualities. What appears doubtful are his social inclinations.

It is true that envy and competition are deeply rooted in

early family life and are latently present in the adult and influence his relationship to other members of society. They have powerful dynamic opponents, however, in the solidarity of the members of a society which is based on identification with each other and a leader. And then there is the low but persistent voice of reason which requires peaceful cooperation. There are significant differences between society and family. Whereas in the family the small children are not expected to contribute to the economic welfare of the group, in society every member is expected to contribute to the survival of the others. In opposition to class struggle is the equally universal principle of the coordination of group interest by compromise and the integration of socially useful activities. The different forms of governments are different methods to achieve this goal. The unresolved envy originating from early experiences of family life is the most potent enemy of this constructive task. Social theories which one-sidedly emphasize only class struggle as the essence of social life and see only the unavoidable imperfections of social mechanisms appeal to this underlying infantile envy and thus activate the disruptive forces in the society. An adequate view of the dynamic structure of society requires the recognition also of the cohesive forces in social life based both on insight and emotions, such as positive identification of the group members with each other and the leader, and constructive, not suppressive, leadership.

One of the most controversial questions of political theory concerns the question: how much government is needed to regulate social activities? Political theorists can be divided into two opposing groups according to their answer to this question. The one type of theory best represented by Plato, Machiavelli, Hobbes, Marx, and Pareto has no trust in the peaceful qualities of human beings and therefore advocates the need for a strong hand no matter whether it is a monarch, a dictator, or an all-powerful political party which keeps in check the unlimited selfishness of the members. Basically, these are the totalitarian theories, and in general they are considered the more realistic. The other group is best represented by Locke, Bentham, and Jefferson, who had a greater trust in enlightened self-interest, in the power of reason. They believed that, given opportunities, people without too much outside interference find the ways and means to coordinate their opposing interests by parliamentary procedures which result in some form of compromise. The first type of theory emphasizes fear as the major factor which keeps people in check; the second theory has greater faith in man's capacity for self-imposed control and allows more individual self-expression.

What can psychiatry contribute to the solution of this fundamental controversy?

First, it contributes recognition of the fact that human nature is not static and predetermined but is pliable and offers a wide range of extremely different combinations. Freud's emphasis upon the importance of early experiences in family life was the first step toward this dynamic concept of human personality, in sharp contrast to the earlier constitutional views most crudely expressed by Lombroso and his school as well as by the racial psychologists such as Chamberlain, Gobineau, and, more recently, Jung. According to these authors, a person's psychological make-up depends primarily upon inherited qualities and his fate is determined by his descent. The congenital criminal of Lombroso, with his characteristic skull structure, protruding jaw and ears and receding forehead, is the crudest example of the view that a person is born criminal, neurotic, psychotic, aggressive, or good-natured not through the influence of his family and social environment but by the genes of the parental cells from which he originated. Freud and his school demonstrated the fallacy of these views by establishing how the emotionally significant events of early life, the whole emotional climate of the family—the relationship between parents and children, and the interrelationship among the children—determined step by step the socially pertinent characteristics of an individual. In the light of the facts unearthed by this type of genetic psychology, the extreme one-sidedness of those views which put exclusive emphasis upon heredity became evident. The new genetic psychology of Freud did not deny the existence of basic hereditary qualities but showed the wide range of evolutionary potentialities of the inherited substratum.

Anthropologists like Kardiner, Linton, Benedict, Mead, Gorer, Kluckholm, and others, by applying psychoanalytic knowledge, show that national characteristics develop primarily under the influence of experiences like those of the child in his family. What makes a German a German, an American an American, a Japanese a Japanese is the intricate effect of factors specific to the Japanese, the American, or the German family. According to anthropologists, racial characteristics are in this respect of little importance. This can be best demonstrated through the American civilization where within two or three generations immigrants from different cultural and ethnic groups have developed a personality type which can be well characterized as American.

The next problem was to establish what determines the typical family attitudes prevailing in a certain culture. Kardiner and Linton were first to emphasize that social organization and social institutions determine parental attitudes and are responsible for the basic personality structure characteristic for members of a culture. Similarly, Ruth Benedict stated that the traditional cultural orientation of a nation as a whole determines the prevailing family attitudes, which in turn again contribute to the personality formation of the child. She has shown that emphasis in the Japanese family upon duty, filial reverence, and observance of a rigid code of behavior can be traced back to the whole structure and history of the Japanese nation, a reflection of a hierarchical feudal system which existed in Japan for many centuries. The ethos of the Japanese family clearly reflects the loyal attitude of the retainer toward his feudal lord. The American personality in many respects is in direct contrast to the Japanese. Nothing is more characteristic of the American than his extreme informality, lack of consistent patterns of behavior, and his resultant adaptability. Whereas the Japanese has a lifelong sense of indebtedness to his parents which he must spend his life in repaying, the American puts emphasis on the concept of the self-made man. Whereas the Japanese self-respect is dependent on how successfully he can live up to the code of revering his predecessors, the American self-respect is based on how successfully he can outstrip the accomplishment of his predecessors. This is most conspicuous in the immigrant family. The father does not master the language and customs of the new culture. His children and their children have to learn ways different from his and his wife's; these children cannot develop reverence for tradition; their trend is away from tradition. Since immigration, until recently, has been a constant feature in the American scene, its influence upon American character cannot easily be exaggerated. The country was founded upon a protest against the Old World and this protesting remained a characteristic feature of the New World.

All these observations, the step-by-step study of individual development by the method of psychoanalysis and the anthropological studies of the different types of family influences prevailing in different cultures, demonstrate the thesis that human nature cannot be considered as a given static structure but something extremely varied and extremely susceptible to psychological influences.

In this view the eternal controversy between the two basic types of political theory appears in a new light. The question itself, whether or not human nature has sufficient social propensities to make parliamentary procedures possible without an all-powerful government, is a pseudo question. The social propensities of man can be changed, increased or decreased by methodical guidance of early child development and later maturation.

The advocates of strong centralized government, however, have another argument more convincing than their mistrust of the social propensities of man. In our present days a potent new need appears on the political scene—the need for social security. Social theorists argue that because of the complexities of modern economic life centralized planning and supervision have become necessary. Otherwise the economic apparatus becomes hopelessly confused, creating uneven distribution of wealth, and periodic depressions and unemployment. The individual has become such an insignificant cogwheel in the large complicated economic mechanism that without governmental protection and guidance he not only *feels* confused but he *is* actually insecure. This accounts for the prevalent insecurity of modern man in this industrial era—for his lack of courage and self-reliance, the decline of his adventurous spirit, and for his longing for a paternalistic government.

According to these theoreticians, social security, particularly that of the weaker members of society, requires an all-pervasive central regulation of economic life by government, the logical end result of which is government ownership and distribution of economic production.

Two great principles oppose each other: individual creativeness, initiative and self-expression, versus security. The proponents of strong central government require a tremendous price for a smooth functioning of our complex society. They would have us sacrifice the most valuable aspect of life, the creative self-expression of the individual. It is for this reason that even ardent advocates of strict suppressive governmental methods support their argument not with claims of desirability but of necessity, because even if people were willing to cooperate, no individual has a comprehensive view of the total socioeconomic picture; therefore, he relies on the guidance of a central government. The proponents of this view like to compare society with the biological organism. In the highly developed multicellular organism, each body cell is dependent upon the functions of all the others and only through a very complex, highly centralized nervous and chemical regulation can life persist.

The conflict between individual security and self-expression is not a pseudo problem but a real one. In our complex industrial civilization it is the crucial problem, the central issue which has divided the world into two great factions. The psychiatrists' contribution to its solution is limited. One fact is certain, that in sacrificing individual self-expression for the sake of greater security achieved by centralized government the coordination of social activities may be improved, but at the same time social conditions will be frozen at the level at which these reforms take place.

Those who think that human inventiveness and creativeness have reached their limits and are satisfied with what we have at present will be inclined to advocate greater security at the cost of less self-expression. Those more enterprising persons who believe in change—in increasing knowledge and the exploration of unknown territories—will be satisfied with less security and will be more interested in freedom for individual development. This consideration is particularly important in our present era of scientific development. All the changes and development of the last three hundred years are ultimately the results of the advancement of scientific knowledge which began in the free atmosphere of the early Renaissance as a reaction against the frozen stability of the Middle Ages. Scientific development, particularly new basic discoveries, requires complete freedom for the scientist to pursue his own curiosities. It is only for the practical application of basic principles which have already been established that science can be blueprinted. The discovery of new knowledge in exploration of the hitherto unknown cannot be centrally planned and organized in advance. Science is the product of the curiosity of the human mind, and only if this curiosity is given free rein can science flourish. Naturally, the same is true for all other creative functions such as art and literature. Nothing demonstrates this better than the rapid development of science, art, and literature in the Renaissance, when man became liberated both socially and spiritually from the rigidity of the feudal system. During these years of the Middle Ages, the security of the people, considering their primitive technical equipment, was relatively great. Their social functions and social place were strictly determined. The serf's life from cradle to grave was secured by the care of his feudal lord. After eight centuries of this kind of stability, the course of history took a turn and the period of adventure started. Man began to explore at first the earth, then the forces of physical nature, and finally his own body and personality. Our present era is but the continuation of the same phase of history which started in the urban areas of Nothern Italy, some five hundred years ago. The question is, are we at the end of this era and must we accept again a rigidly blueprinted society for another eight hundred years?

It is not for psychiatrists to answer these questions. Psychiatry and anthropology have demonstrated that human nature can be influenced, that peaceful and creative qualities can be fostered by one type of education and martial aggressive qualities by another. The inclination toward a rigid centralization and organization of social life stems primarily from insecurity. This insecurity does not stem from the complexities of modern society alone but from the constant threat of war. There is little doubt that the regulation of the social mechanism does not require such far-reaching suppression of individual expression as is aimed at by the totalitarian systems. Only external danger, the continuous threat of war, necessitates a rigid suppression of individual freedoms. Those thinkers who like the analogy between society and the body should be reminded that the internal economic processes of the organisms, the vegetative functions, have a much greater local autonomy and are much less centrally governed than those functions of the organism concerned with the relationship to the external world. This comes to expression in the differentiation between cerebrospinal and the autonomic nervous system. The autonomic nervous system, as its name shows, though connected with the central government has a relatively great independence. This is particularly true for the peripheral so-called intrinsic ganglia of the guts and the heart, which function like small autonomous local governments although their activity receives regulatory influences from the higher centers. Only the voluntary behavior of the organism which concerns its external policies is under strict centralized government. I do not mention this because I think that the analogy between society and organism can be carried very far but only to show that those who claim a biological foundation for strictly centralized government have not a clear-cut support for their thesis even in biology.

There are many possible forms of organization. Biological organism and most human societies are based in many ways on diametrically opposite principles. Most human societies are characterized by the emphasis upon the individual. An exception is the totalitarian state, which tries to imitate biological organisms. The cells of an organism completely renounce their independence and live only through and for the total organism. In most human societies, social institutions serve the interest of the individual by making his struggle for existence require less effort, thus saving energy which can be spent for creative activities. Without the latter, life in human society would become similar to that in an insect state. The insect state represents a transition between society and biological organisms. The individual members depend upon the functions of the other members and need even their bodily secretions for their own survival. In such a highly organized society, the security of the members may be great but their activities are reduced to mere vegetation and propagation. The valid question arises, whether life in such a well-organized and standardized society would still be worth living.

We must stop here and realize that we are in danger of confusing two issues: the type of world we want to live in, and how scientific understanding of man and society can contribute to achieve this world. It must have become clear by now that the type of society which serves the person best and allows him the fullest expression of his individual creative abilities is threatened by the present increased need for security. For the sake of greater security, man appears to be inclined to sacrifice all those specifically human values which make life worth living. Whatever science could contribute to increasing security without sacrificing individuality and free expression would help to resolve this great dilemma of our times. In a world from which the threat of war could be eliminated, the need to sacrifice individuality for security would be greatly diminished.

What can psychiatry contribute toward a more peaceful world?

In theory, at least, a group of psychiatrists and social scientists could work out a blueprint of education by which a peaceful, productive, cooperative type of human material would be produced. How such a blueprint could be realized is the crucial question.

The same facts of anthropology which demonstrate the pliability of human nature should also warn us against exalted hopes. They show us that the emotional orientation of people and the social structure in which this develops are inseparable. They constitute an organic unit and can only be changed together. Psychiatry has developed methods suitable to influence an individual, but it is beyond the scope of psychiatry to influence the ideology and attitudes prevailing within a whole culture. It is not psychiatrists but parents who influence the child's development, and parental attitudes again are determined by the total culture. This should warn us also against future projects of reeducating other nations by introducing to them attitudes which do not spring from their own cultural soil. To make warriors of a nation of peaceful agricultural settlers without changing their whole socioeconomic system is just as impossible as exterminating the warlike spirit of nomadic hunters whose existence depends upon fostering martial qualities in their children. We must conclude, then, that it lies beyond the scope of psychiatry to influence the ideology and attitudes prevailing within whole cultures. The application of psychiatric principles to rearing a generation with an emotional outlook conducive for peace, even in the framework of a single nation, appears an immense task. On a world scale it is an even more Utopian goal. It would first of all require universal agreement as to the type of the desirable emotional orientation to be achieved, and only if the same goal were adopted all over the world would such measures contribute to world peace.

There is only one fact which brings a ray of hope into this gloomy perspective. I refer to cultural change. Family attitudes are determined by the social configuration prevailing in a culture and are transmitted from generation to generation by tradition. Traditional attitudes, particularly the ways of child rearing change more slowly than does the social configuration itself. This brings about a discrepancy between existing social conditions and traditional attitudes. The latter belong to the past and lag behind the actual conditions in a changing society. This lag between existing conditions and social attitudes inherited from the past can easily be observed in our present era because of the rapidity of social change.

While the cultural lag may manifest itself in various ways in different nations, there are certain discrepancies between out-moded attitudes and changed conditions which today are universal. In none of the existing cultures has man yet succeeded in adapting his attitude to his rapidly acquired technological mastery of nature. Now, in a time of potential plenty, he still lives according to the law of the jungle where the scarcity of food makes one alternative: to kill or to be killed. He still needs to secure himself against the greed and domination of other nations in a time in which the unhampered use of technological knowledge could create plenty for all. Although he is potentially rich and secure, not through exploiting others but because of his immense capacity for exploiting nature, he still covets the riches of others and must protect his own property from the greed of others. He has to arm himself; he must use technology primarily for military defence and destruction. He therefore cherishes primarily his political and military sovereignty instead of the real sovereignty of his person, his right to be himself in the higher aspects of life. He is ready to sacrifice his spiritual freedom as an individual and trust his fate to the rule of autocratic governments and leaders because he is afraid of being attacked and because he believes that he can prosper only by subjugating his neighbors. Although his mastery over nature alone could make him secure, man has not yet acquired confidence in his own power over nature and so he still wants to dominate his fellow man as a means of security.

Cultural lag can slow down social change, but not prevent it. In our present era, the cultural lag consists in the fact that man has not yet waked up to the fact that the technical mastery of nature makes him secure and that he does not need to subjugate others to increase his own welfare and security. The psychiatrists' function is to counteract the cultural lag by hastening the intellectual and emotional adaptation to existing conditions. This requires an increased knowledge of personality formation. New knowledge will come from further, more precise study of what may be called the emotional structure of the whole family. In the past studies, the center of attention was the child as he is influenced by his relationship to the members of the family; the understanding of the total configuration of the family still wants further investigation. This field may properly be called the psychodynamics of the family. The second part of the problem, the sociodynamics of the family, is concerned with the question of how family attitudes are determined by the larger social configuration, by social structure, tradition, geography, and history. This field is still almost virgin territory.

Our present psychiatric knowledge is restricted to helping the neurotic individual and to some extent to influencing the education of the child. This knowledge and these skills have no immediate influence on the course of world affairs. It is true that we have learned a great deal in the last fifty years about the motivation of man's behavior and that we have learned how to apply this knowledge to the individual with fair success. To influence the growing generations within one nation through psychiatry is a long-term project; to influence the interrelationship of nations will take even longer. What we must be aware of in this connection are the tremendous gaps in our present knowledge. The emphasis must therefore be on further research in this new aspect of social psychiatry and anthropology.

All this will require time and peace. We are engaged in a desperate race between the development of our scientific knowledge of society on the one hand and the rapid deterioration of international relationships on the other. Nothing would be more fateful than to put our faith in the hope that with our present psychiatric and sociological knowledge and facilities we can bring about world peace. It must be maintained by other means. In the meantime, we must endeavor to develop a valid science of sociodynamics which in the future may contribute to maintaining peace and assuring a more reasonable relationship between nations, not by force but by a gradual change of social institutions and the emotional orientation of the people.

METHUSELAH: MYTH OR PROMISE

By David Seegal, M.D.*

LIFE IS SWEET, but is it long enough for Man? In the preface to *Back to Methuselah,* Bernard Shaw bemoans the fact that "Even our oldest men do not live long enough: they are, for all the purposes of high civilization, mere children when they die; and our Prime Ministers, though rated as mature, divide their time between the golf course and the treasury bench in Parliament."

Adam and Eve and Methuselah and his family are unique in their long flight toward earthly immortality. The 969 years of Methuselah's life stand out in contrast to the outer limit of one hundred years for modern man. The chill hand of scientific critique has pointed a questioning finger at Methuselah's purported age. For the purposes of the present discussion we will disregard such skepticism and allow Methuselah's longevity to become our romantic ideal.

The search to lengthen the span of life has occupied the mind of man since recorded history. It is well at the outset to draw attention to two apparently separate factors which influence longevity. The first of these concerns the control of the natural aging process which proceeds independent

* Now Professor of Medicine, College of Physicians and Surgeons, Columbia University and Director, Columbia Research Service, Goldwater Memorial Hospital, New York.

of disease. We know little about this in man, but some interesting experiments in animals may lead to a new understanding. The second factor concerns the control of those diseases which, unchecked, cripple or kill man. Untreated, such diseases as diabetes mellitus, pernicious anemia, pellagra, and syphilis interrupt the normal skein of longevity.

Our knowledge of the natural aging mechanism in the human is largely limited to statistics concerning the duration of life. In 1975 over 18 million of our population, having reached 65 or more, will then present challenges to our statesmen, economists, and physicians. Figure 1, from Dublin, Latka, and Spiegelman, *Length of Life,* shows the increase in the average length of life from ancient to modern times. Contrast the life expectancy of 22 years at the time of Christ to the present average of 66.7 years. Particularly striking is the rise from 49 years in 1900 to 66 years in 1946.

The recent popular literature contains references to methods purporting to postpone expected old age. We are aware of Voronov's statements that youth might be reclaimed by the transplantation of the sex glands of lower animals to man. These claims have not stood the test of scientific examination. More recently, Bogomolets, a president of the Ukrainian Academy of Sciences, described a serum effective in the prevention and treatment of a whole host of diseases. The serum was obtained from an animal which had previously been injected with human bone marrow or spleen. Bogomolets reported that a series of very small injections of this serum would mitigate arteriosclerosis and retard the aging process. Our examination of the available papers published by this worker fails to disclose evidence to support his claims. Bogomolets died rather unexpectedly at the age of 63.

Scientific investigators have usually studied lower forms of life in order to obtain information of benefit to man. In this way they have learned much about the natural life of plants and animals. They have then proceeded to influence this "natural life" in a variety of experiments, some of which we shall shortly describe.

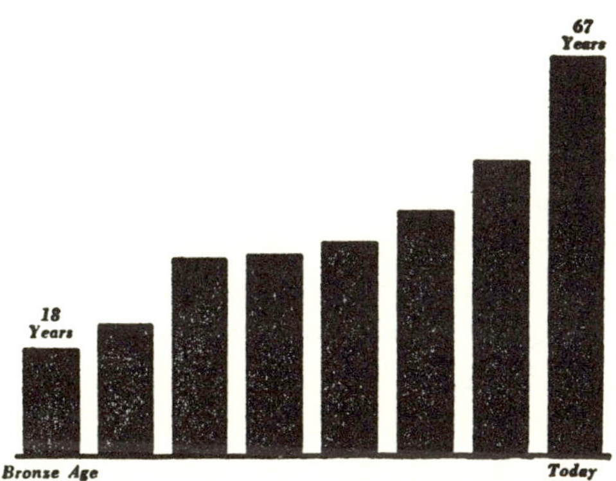

FIGURE 1. INCREASE IN THE AVERAGE LENGTH OF LIFE FROM ANCIENT TO MODERN TIMES

From L. I. Dublin and Others, *Length of Life,* rev. ed., New York, Ronald Press, 1949.

May I first discuss the "natural life" of some representative plants and animals. The glow, if not the light of immortality, has been thrown on single-celled plants, since they reproduce continuously by cell division. Rolleston has stated that,

> In the simplest forms of animal life, the protozoa, which consist of a single cell and so stand in the same relation to man that a brick does to a city, multiplication occurs by fission, or division into two halves, and as there are now two cells instead of one and no vestige of a corpse, the organism, as Weismann first insisted, is immortal. . . . If the protozoa are, accidents apart, immortal, why is it that animals much higher in the scale never are?

Rolleston suggests that this cannot be realized because the cells become part of a larger differentiated whole. "In the higher walks of the animal kingdom rejuvenation of the constituent cells is thus rendered much more difficult or impossible, and the problem of senescence must be regarded as the penalty for the high degree of individualization entailed in the complicated mechanism of higher animals and man."

Some perennial plants, such as the giant redwood trees, have lived forty centuries. In contrast, the animal kingdom has a relatively short span of life. According to Howard, "The true insects . . . are extremely fugitive individuals . . . so fugitive that they die before it seems possible that they are old." As far as is known the signs of wear and tear, and thus of aging, are not manifested in the insect world. An exception is said to be the worker bee, the indomitable woman of the hive, whose wings become fragmented and whose hair is lost before death.

The life span of vertebrates, the back-boned animals, though much greater than that of insects, falls far short of that of most plants. Todd has stated that, "with few exceptions, among mammals, birds, reptiles and perhaps fish, 50 years is the probable limit of vertebrate life. The majority, no matter what their size, reach the extreme of survival at between 25 and 35 years."

Todd has suggested that, "the potential life of most mammals is naturally controlled by the state of the teeth: when these wear away or fall out starvation or attack quickly closes the record." The life span of modern man, protected by his dentist for mastication if not for combat, may be considerably greater than 50 years. Dublin, the elder, has stated that, "by some inexorable law, still to be discovered and clarified, nature has allotted to man a life span of about 100 years. But very few lives complete this span."

To illustrate the wide variation in duration of life among living things, consider the amoeba which, in a sense, may be considered immortal; the redwood tree, which has already lived 3500 years; the baby Venus, who can look forward to 70 years; and the May fly, whose stay on earth is limited to but one or two days.

The physical and mental characteristics usually associated with different stages of aging are not invariable concomitants. Frank has reminded us "that aging or senescence occurs frequently in men and women who, chronologically speaking, are relatively young; likewise, delayed aging is found among men and women of advanced chronological age who exhibit good health and few, if any, signs of impairment or enfeeblement."

It is unfortunate that we are ignorant of the mechanism responsible for that bizarre condition in man in which the velocity of aging is highly accelerated. This rare clinical picture is called progeria, which means "prematurely old." Figure 2 shows a 17-year-old youth seen by Gilford. You will note how senile the small body appears. The skull seems large because the facial bones are underdeveloped. A few bits of downy hair are visible. The skin is wrinkled and flabby. A number of findings were present which suggested heart and blood-vessel damage. This was confirmed at the death of this 17-year-old boy, since the aorta, the large vessel carrying blood from the heart, was so calcareous (arteriosclerotic) that the openings to both the heart muscle arteries were blocked. This degree of arteriosclerosis is frequently associated with adult life and not with youth. Talbot has reported a case of progeria in a boy who died at 7½ years of age with advanced arteriosclerosis. In fact, the effects of the arteriosclerosis caused his death. Although these cases have stimulated considerable thought, they have not as yet yielded information to explain the mechanism of the premature aging and arteriosclerosis.

One fact concerning aging in man is generally accepted. This is the genetic transmissibility of the potential for longevity. Long-lived families are known to all of us. There seems little doubt from studies in the common fruit fly (*Drosophila melanogaster*) that duration of life under controlled conditions is often associated with differences in subtypes. Thus the short-winged variety of the fruit fly uniformly has a shorter life span than the usual normal-winged variety. This difference is unrelated to the environment.

The transmissibility of the capacity for longevity in man has usually taken place by chance mating. It is reasonable to conclude from present data that selective breeding would increase the strains of longevity in the population after many, many generations.

Two pieces of experimental work have recently come to light which promise to increase our understanding of the mechanism of "natural" aging and its control. Herbert Evans, who has made signal contributions in the field of endocrinology, has reported the maintenance of a prolonged period of growth, youthfulness, and health in the rat by the injection of a hormone, a pure product of the anterior lobe of the pituitary gland. With his associates, Evans treated adult rats with this material. The animals were about 200 days old and weighed approximately one-half pound at the start of the experiment. When they were over 400 days old, equivalent to the last trimester of life in man, they had received 37 treatments and had doubled their weight. The treated rats appeared surprisingly young, robust, and active. The increase in stature and tissue growth were in the tradition of youthful development. There was no excess fat, and careful examination of the rats failed to disclose the abnormalities expected in the aged animal. The organs, although large, were well proportioned. The bones were of particular interest. They were characteristic of the young animal and had continued to grow to the end of the experiment. In contrast, the bones, as well as the other tissues of the control, untreated rats were stigmatized by the changes of old age.

The second piece of experimental work which may point a way to a better and longer life for man is concerned with a study in nutrition. The beginnings of this work go back twenty-five years to observations made in a fish hatchery. Dr. Clive M. McCay, then a Research Fellow at Yale, was assigned to study the growth of trout with the idea of reducing the cost of feeding them. He found to his surprise that if the rations of the trout were cut down, they grew more slowly and lived longer. McCay then proceeded to investigate the influence of diet on longevity in the rodent. He found that when rats are maintained on a well-balanced but low-protein, low-calory diet, their growth is retarded. However, these rats live much longer than their control litter mates who have been given supplementary rations. For instance, the controls live only 2 to 3 years at the utmost, whereas the underfed rats usually live well over 3 years. The eldest died just short of 4 years of age, comparable to 140 years of life for man. These rodent Methuselahs remained healthy, vigorous and fertile to within a few weeks of death. Recently, Rorty has summarized these data for the layman in a lucid and interesting article in *Harper's Magazine,* "The Thin Rats Bury the Fat Rats." This title summarizes McCay's major experience. It is of interest that the over-all results at the Cornell nutrition laboratory also reveal that the female rats generally bury the male rats. Dr. McCay tells me that he considers the female better equipped than the male rat for longevity. Certainly the vital statistics for humans point in a similar direction.

Figure 3, taken from a report by McCay and Crowell, shows photographs of two rats, both 890 days old. At this age the normal rat on a nonrestricted diet may be said to be old. This is borne out by the withered appearance of the rat on the left. Contrast this senile rodent with the rat shown on the right who has lived on a well-balanced but low-calory diet to this same age. Although the latter is smaller than the other rat, he appears youthful and normal.

Figure 4 is a photograph of two of McCay's rats which were fed a well-balanced, but low-calory diet for 1320 days. They have many of the earmarks of senility but these rats have long outlived their free-eating litter mates. Furthermore, these chronologically old rats are reported to have been active, well spirited, good-humored and fertile.

It is hazardous to conclude that the results of animal experimentation may be directly related to human experience. Nevertheless, it is of more than passing interest that the statistics compiled by the Life Insurance Companies indicate clearly that the *thin men bury the fat men*. Even mild obesity is said to foreshadow a shortening of the life expectancy.

The few facts known concerning the experimental prolongation of life in animals in the absence of disease may point out some directions in the study of man's longevity. It is apparent that one should first choose one's ancestors with care. If that is not possible perhaps a better control of endocrine and nutritional balance will achieve desirable results. The road ahead for this and other experimental work of a similar nature may be long and difficult, albeit rewarding.

The part which diseases play in limiting longevity is clearly defined. The scourge of acute infectious diseases decimated the populations of the Middle Ages. A walk through New England graveyards of the last century indicates the difficulty of reaching full maturity at that time, because of the death-dealing blows of dysentery, pneumonia, diphtheria, scarlet fever, cholera, phthisis, and childbed fever. Even as late as 1918, 21,000,000 people died in

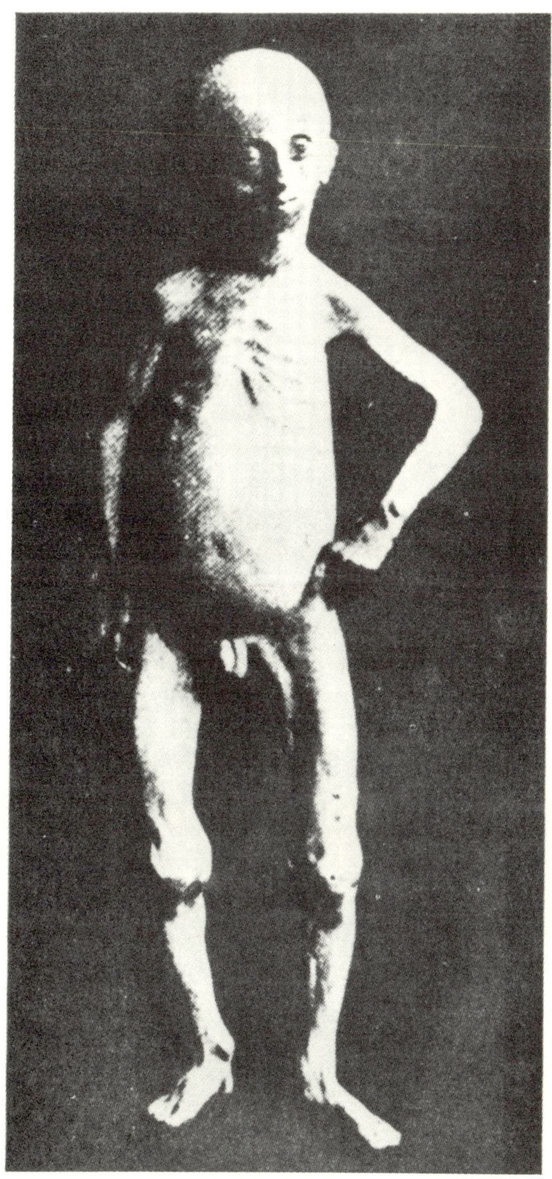

FIGURE 2. PROGERIA

From Hastings Gilford, "Progeria: a Form of Senilism," *Practitioner,* 73:188, 1904.

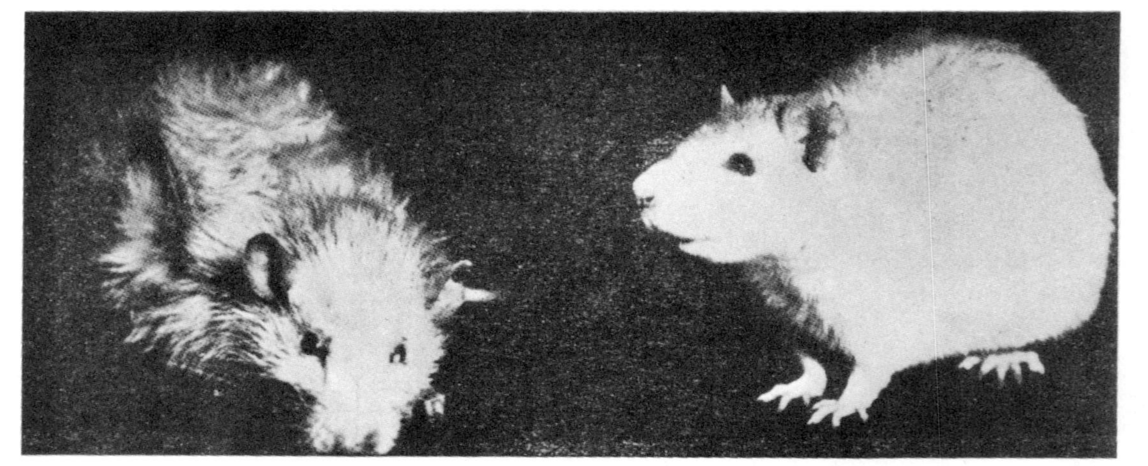

FIGURE 3. TWO RATS 890 DAYS OF AGE

The animal on the left was maintained on a normal diet, the one on the right was given a well-balanced, but low calory diet throughout the period. (After McCay and Crowell)

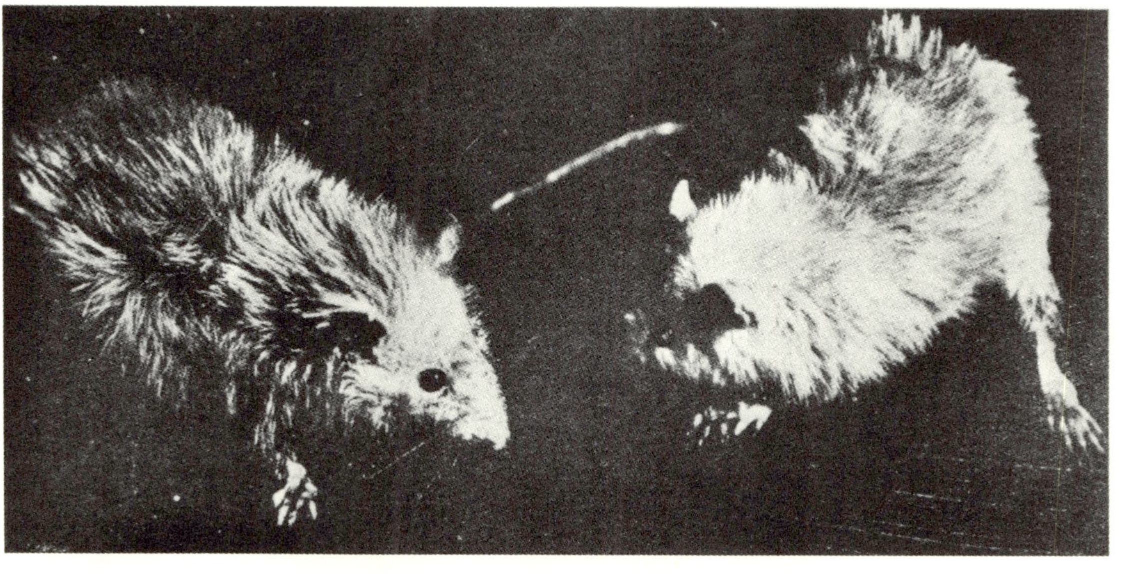

Figure 4. Rats on a Restricted Diet

These animals are alive at the age of 1320 days, which is approximately twice the normal expected duration of life for rats of this strain. (After McCay and Crowell)

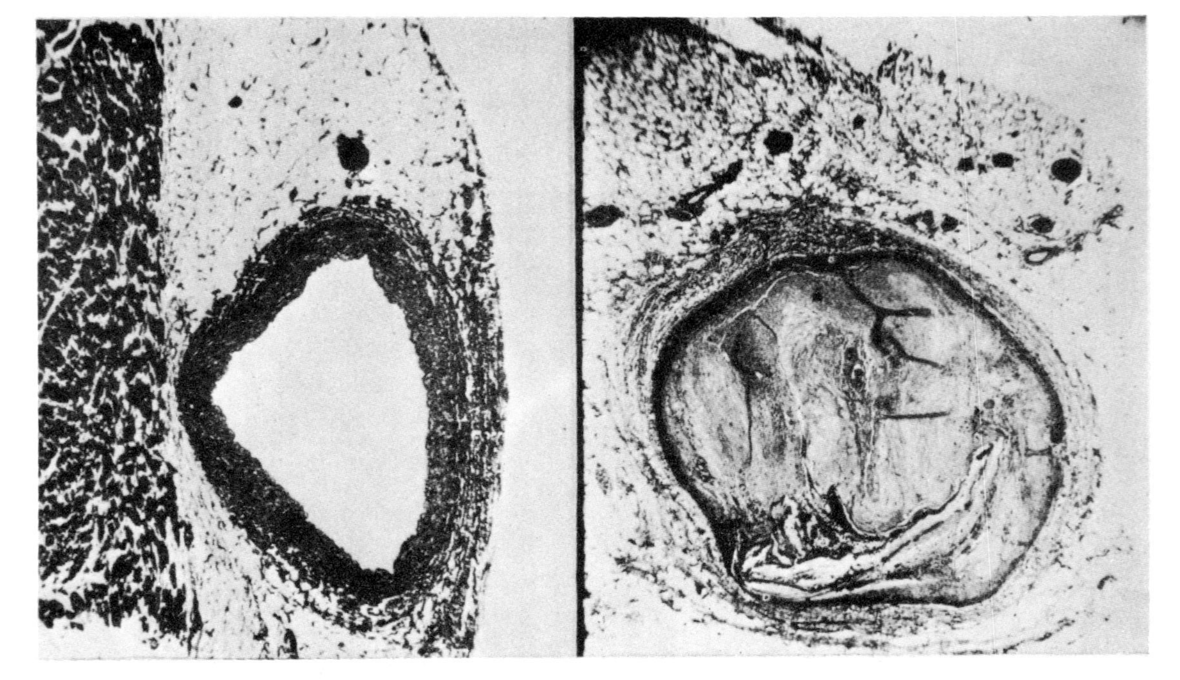

Figure 5. Coronary Arteries of Two Males, One 76 Years Old and the Other 33

(Courtesy of Dr. Bevans)

the influenza epidemic. But nature's curtain opened a little further and we came upon the era of antibiotics. It is largely through our increasing control of acute infectious diseases that the average life expectancy of women has been extended to 70.28 years.

Nature's curtain, however, has not opened wide enough as yet to allow us to gain the tools to prevent and control many of the long-term or chronic illnesses. Although medical science has made considerable headway in this difficult field, man's life is foreshortened today because of our inability to effectively meet the challenges of such diseases as high blood pressure, hardening of the arteries, and cancer.

In order to learn more about chronic disease it has been necessary to differentiate the features of the life-destroying diseases of middle age from the characteristics of the aging process. Stieglitz has emphasized the difficulties inherent in this subject. Frank has stated the problem in this manner: "The issue becomes sharply focused upon the possibility of distinguishing between the cumulative, physiological involutions that inevitably take place in all individuals as they grow older, and pathological changes that occur in aging individuals as the result of adverse environmental conditions."

The possibility of confusing these two mechanisms is well illustrated by the experience of plant pathologists. Early horticulturists, in characterizing the different stages in the development of plants, were wont to ascribe certain structural changes to "age degeneration." These defects were visible to the naked eye. Petunia leaves developed variegated areas of discoloration; tomato plant leaves exhibited light spots; and tobacco plant leaves became discolored, mottled, and stunted. However, when modern microbiological techniques became available, in many cases specific viruses were isolated from these so-called "aged" plants. When the studies were completed it was possible to conclude that often the plant defects were due to an infectious agent. If this analogy could be transferred to the human, some of the so-called stigmata of age degeneration in man might eventually be shown to result from specific diseases.

Some scientists have held that the guillotines and reapers' scythes of hardening of the arteries or high blood pressure represent the summary implements in the aging process. But this does not seem valid since the blades on the scythes of such other chronic diseases as diabetes mellitus and pernicious anemia have been dulled by medical research so that these illnesses are now largely controlled. It is pertinent, therefore, to consider disease as an unnatural bedfellow of the aging process.

Let us examine the relationship which exists between chronological age and arteriosclerosis. In the past, arteriosclerosis was considered a direct concomitant of age. In the main, this is true, but the exceptions are intriguing and numerous, and possibly point to the Achilles heel of the problem. Dr. Bevans, of Montego Bay, has provided me with Figure 5, which shows sections of the coronary or heart arteries of two males, one 33 and the other 76 years of age. That of the 33-year-old man shows extensive arteriosclerosis in contrast to that of the elderly gentleman which is free of the process. Some of us have come to the notion that the lesions of arteriosclerosis represent a disorder in fat metabolism. We do not consider this disease an inevitable concomitant of the aging process.

Ivy has taken an optimistic view concerning the ultimate control of arteriosclerosis. He has presented a series of observations to strengthen "the view that something can be done about arteriosclerosis." His thoughts run in these directions: About a third of a large series of individuals over the age of 80 were shown to have a remarkably small amount of arteriosclerosis. It was, therefore, impossible to relate the degree of hardening of the arteries directly to the duration of life. Arteriosclerosis was found to be more prevalent in the male. This might be a lead for fruitful investigation. For unknown reasons, arteriosclerosis of the heart arteries is more common in white persons than in Negroes. Arteriosclerosis is distributed irregularly in the blood vessels throughout the body. The need for investigation of this vagary is obvious. Arteriosclerosis occurs with greater frequency and intensity in certain other pathological states such as kidney disease and diabetes mellitus. It is of interest that these diseases have in common a high content of cholesterol, a fatty substance, in the blood. It is now possible to produce a close counterpart of human arteriosclerosis in a variety of animals, including the dog, by the administration of an excess quantity of cholesterol, the fatty substance mentioned above. It has been said that the Chinese living in China have much less arteriosclerosis than the average American. A number of observers have correlated this finding with the low-fat, low-protein, low-calory diets of the Chinese.

This discussion concerning arteriosclerosis indicates that its effects need no longer be considered a reflection of normal aging. It also is meant to suggest that sufficient clues and experimental evidence have appeared to loosen the strings on its cloak of inevitability. Nevertheless, arteriosclerosis is still one of our chief uncontrolled chronic diseases. In order that you may not draw the conclusion that our knowledge concerning other chronic diseases is similarly limited I should like to turn to an account of the progress which has been made since the turn of the century in the control of the long-term illnesses in man. This study was undertaken with Drs. Colcher, Duane, and Wertheim. The results of their survey have led us to an optimistic attitude.

For the purposes of this discussion may we define chronic illness as a state requiring medical, surgical, or ancillary care for periods of six months or longer. The derivation of the word chronic is from the Greek word, *Chronos,* meaning time. Other criteria for classification have not proved as satisfactory as the factor of time.

Various surveys show that about one out of six people in the United States has a chronic disease. This figure is misleading, however, since the term disease does not necessarily imply illness. Although many persons age 25 have some degree of arteriosclerosis, the great majority of them do not show signs of this illness. In later years, unless the disease comes under control, many members of this group may be expected to develop impairment of efficiency of the heart, brain, or legs due to progressive damage to the arteries.

A common misconception is that chronic diseases are confined to the aged. On the contrary, about 16 percent of patients with chronic illnesses are under 25 years of age, and about 50 percent are below the age of 45. It is thus seen that chronic disease may disable many individuals in the prime of life and thus compromise their expected longevity.

The brilliant results attained in the treatment of acute infectious diseases with modern chemotherapeutic agents such as the sulfonamides, streptomycin, penicillin, aureomycin, and terramycin have overshadowed the less dramatic progress made in the control of chronic illness. However, when the latter is examined, it is apparent that medical science has made considerable headway in this difficult field. Many chronic diseases which brought death or disabling illness 30 years ago are now controlled. For example, with early diagnosis and adequate treatment, *pelagra, amebiasis, hyperthyroidism,* and certain *congenital heart defects* can be cured.

Hyperthyroidism is a metabolic disorder caused by overactivity of the thyroid gland. This sits below the Adam's apple and encircles the front of the windpipe like a small horseshoe. The symptoms of hyperthyroidism are familiar. If the subject is a young woman, she is apt to attract more than the usual attention because of her prominent eyes and animated actions and conversation. The thyroid gland is often visibly enlarged, and a tremor or shaking of the fingers is present. Because of this disturbance, the lady may frequently drop the dish she is drying or make mistakes at typewriting she has not made before. This often leads to criticism, recrimination, and tears. Since the overactivity of the thyroid gland sharply increases body heat production, the subject is frequently uncomfortable in the summer and welcomes the frigidity of winter with silken disdain.

This disease occasionally runs a long course before it is recognized. The most satisfactory present method of treatment is surgical removal of a large part of the gland. In good hands, this results in cure in all but a few cases. The recent introduction of thiouracil and related compounds and of radioactive iodine for the treatment of hyperthyroidism has produced encouraging results, but it is too early to draw a final conclusion concerning their effectiveness in the long run.

Congenital heart defects result from a disorderly growth of the heart during embryological evolution. Some of these defects are of such a slight degree that they cause no trouble. Others, however, prevent the heart from fulfilling its responsibility as the master pump of the body. A variety of symptoms and signs appear, including the cyanosis, the blueness, which has recently been so much publicized. This may be due to a defect which prevents a proper amount of blood returning from the outer body to reach the lungs for oxygenation. Or the blueness may result from an imperfect wall between the right and left side of the heart, thus allowing unoxygenated blue blood to be mixed with the outgoing red blood. Brilliant researches and surgical performances in Boston and Baltimore have resulted in transforming hundreds of chronically disabled heart invalids into happy, care-free children.

Other chronic illnesses, such as *pernicious anemia, diabetes mellitus* and *syphilis* can be largely controlled.

Diabetes mellitus is characterized by an inability on the part of the individual to utilize sugar properly. Banting's discovery of insulin in 1922 has revolutionized the outlook for patients with this chronic illness.

Pernicious anemia is a deficiency disease in which the total number of red blood cells is sharply decreased. The mortality in this chronic illness in the past was almost 100 percent. In 1926 Minot and Murphy reported that the ingestion of one-half pound of liver each day controlled this disease. This has been amply confirmed. Since that time liver extract, stomach extract, folic acid, and vitamin B_{12} have produced favorable results. If diagnosis of the disease is made early, and if the treatment is rigorously maintained, the patient with pernicious anemia may look forward to a long and useful life.

Syphilis, a former scourge of mankind whose initial damage to the body is so slight, may later produce devastating injury to the heart, blood vessels, and brain. With proper preventive medical control and adequate treatment with penicillin and adjuvants, many cases of syphilis are forestalled and others are favorably modified.

Since the advances in the treatment of chronic diseases have occurred chiefly within the past 30 years, it is reasonable to view with optimism the possibility of further early progress. In fact, it was necessary to revise this manuscript to keep up with the recent reports of the advances in the treatment of rheumatoid arthritis and allied conditions by cortisone and ACTH.

In addition to the chronic diseases which are cured or largely controlled by early diagnosis and adequate treatment, there is a considerable group of other long-term illnesses which may be partially controlled. My colleagues and I have recently reviewed this matter and were able to list a group of 37 chronic illnesses which are partially controlled. The therapeutic measures, while not curative in this group, produce more than mere symptomatic relief. I propose to discuss briefly about five of the diseases listed in this category.

In *Addison's disease* the adrenal gland is damaged. As the process continues the patient becomes weak and the skin often darkens. In later stages vomiting, collapse, and death may occur. Dr. Loeb, at the Presbyterian Hospital in 1932, found that the sodium or salt content of the blood of these patients was sharply lowered. When a large amount of sodium chloride was given to the patients their well-being returned and life was prolonged. Since that time various preparations containing important chemicals of the adrenal cortex have been used successfully in this condition.

Portal cirrhosis of the liver, often called alcoholic cirrhosis, is not an uncommon chronic disease. Patients may have this disorder for years without manifesting any outward symptoms. When large areas of the specialized liver tissue are replaced by scar tissue, the blood in the abdominal cavity has difficulty finding its way back through the pinched liver blood channels. Among other symptoms, the patient may then develop fluid in his abdominal cavity. Fifteen years ago the great majority of patients who reached this stage of the disease were not expected to survive more than four to six months. But, in 1936, Dr. Patek and his associates, at the Columbia Research Division of the Goldwater Memorial Hospital, introduced the concept that the development of cirrhosis of the liver was only indirectly related to the high consumption of alcohol. These workers held to the belief that the frequent occurrence of low food consumption by the alcoholic played the chief role in the development of portal cirrhosis. Subsequent animal experimentation supports the thesis that a diminished food intake, particularly of protein, leads to cirrhosis in some lower animals. At any rate, Patek and his group have demonstrated that a highly nutritious regimen with vitamin supplements contributes to an increase in the expected longevity of individuals with severe cirrhosis of the liver. Recently other adjuvants to this treatment have been introduced. Among these are the administration of human serum albumin or special liver extracts and surgical methods to allow portions of the blood to by-pass the liver.

The effect of multiple procedures is seen in the efforts that have led to the achievement of partial control of *pulmonary tuberculosis*. Combinations of early diagnosis, sanitarium regimens, methods to produce lung rest (such as compression of the lung by inserting air into the chest cage, or giving complete lung rest by the use of the alternating pressure chamber of Barach), surgical procedures, and streptomycin in selected cases have favorably modified the natural course of this illness. The death rate for tuberculosis in 1947 was less than one fifth that at the turn of the century.

Rheumatic fever is one of the common diseases of childhood and is the chief cause of heart disease in this age group. The migratory inflammation of the joints, though temporarily disabling, leaves no aftermath and is, therefore, of little importance. The tragedy of the disease lies in the associated inflammation in the three layers of the heart. The initial heart damage may be slight, but since rheumatic fever has a great tendency to repeat itself in the same individual the additional effect of one inflammatory attack after another often leads to serious crippling of the heart. We now know, through the work of Coburn, that rheumatic fever is initiated by a hemolytic streptococcus infection. Any method which would prevent hemolytic streptococcus infection would, *pari passu,* prevent further bouts of rheumatic fever. Reports from four clinics indicate that the prophylactic administration of sulfonamides significantly decreases the expected incidence of hemolytic streptococcus infections in children with rheumatic heart disease. This in turn reduces the calculated expectancy for rheumatic recurrence in the same groups. Experiments are now underway to determine the possible usefulness of penicillin given by mouth in place of the sulfonamides. Cortisone, or ACTH, appears to ameliorate this disease.

Rheumatoid arthritis is a distant cousin of rheumatic fever. It is chiefly a disease of adults. Unlike rheumatic fever, the joint inflammation in rheumatoid arthritis is persistent and may progress to destruction of the joint. Heart involvement, on the other hand, is an unusual finding in this disease. An extraordinary list of substances have been tested in the treatment of rheumatoid arthritis but until recently, rest and gold salts seemed to be the most effective agents. Those who have read Laurence's and Kaempffert's reports of the Mayo Clinic experience with cortisone and ACTH are well aware of the fact that either of these substances, cortisone a product of the adrenal gland, or ACTH, a substance from the pituitary gland which stimulates the adrenal gland, will produce an almost miraculous change in the condition of the patient with rheumatoid arthritis. Patients with swollen joints who have been bedridden for months or years walk up and down steps with moderate alacrity 48 hours following the onset of treatment. There are two drawbacks to this form of therapy. The one is the necessity for continued treatment. Otherwise a rapid recurrence of symptoms develops. The second drawback has to do with the possible development of unfavorable symptoms associated with hyperactivity of the adrenal glands.

Let us now consider some of the chronic diseases whose course, in the main, is uncontrolled by medical science. Arteriosclerosis (hardening of the arteries), hypertension (elevated blood pressure), or malignant tumors probably affect the majority of persons who are ill of the uncontrolled chronic diseases. You are acquainted with the increased tempo of research in regard to the nature of cancer. Early diagnosis, surgery, and radiotherapy have made inroads on the devastation wrought by this scourge.

Before further discussion of arteriosclerosis and hypertension may I make some general remarks about heart disease, which is recognized as the present chief killer of mankind. Too often a pessimistic view is taken by the layman with regard to affections of this organ. On the contrary, a review of the progress made in the control of those diseases which compromise the heart is indeed encouraging. Figure 6 attempts to present this point of view in graphic form. In the center is a romantic drawing of the heart. Surrounding this figure are the names of eight diseases which are chiefly responsible for heart disease. You will note that an arrow extends from each name towards the heart and that six out of eight of these arrows' heads are blunted and turned away from the heart. This is to indicate the increasing medical control of diphtheria, hyperthyroidism, congenital heart disease, syphilis, rheumatic fever, and bacterial endocarditis. In two instances, arteriosclerosis and hypertension, the arrows' heads plunge deeply into the heart to indicate our lack of control.

Diphtheria may be prevented or treated by appropriate

immunological methods. Surgical procedures control hyperthyroidism and some congenital heart defects. An adequate public health program with the aid of antibiotics is minimizing the harmful effects of syphilis on the heart. At least 80 percent of patients with subacute bacterial endocarditis are now cured of the infection. Optimistic reports have appeared indicating that chemoprophylaxis may prevent the harmful hemolytic streptococcus infections in the patient with rheumatic fever and thus prevent further damage to the heart. Favorable reports concerning the use of ACTH and cortisone in this disease are now at hand.

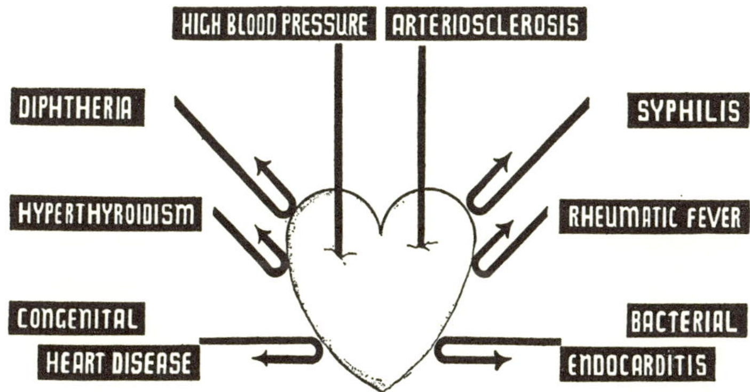

FIGURE 6. PROGRESS IN THE CONTROL OF HEART DISEASE

The arrow points deflected from the surface of the heart symbolize the increasing medical control of six diseases responsible for heart damage. The two arrows plunging into the heart symbolize the uncontrolled afflictions of the heart.

There are thus left only two other major causes of heart disease, arteriosclerosis and hypertension. Brisk research work now under way is leading to the increased understanding of the nature of these abnormalities. We have already discussed some studies on arteriosclerosis. The investigations in hypertension have been concerned with the elaboration of substances in the body which raise blood pressure, the influence of nervous impulses on the maintenance of normal and abnormal blood pressures, and finally, the effect of restricted diets on pressure levels. The fruits of these researches have led to operations which effectively reduce the blood pressure in a small group of patients and to the introduction of salt-poor diets, or a rice diet, which mitigate the high blood pressure in some patients. This brief summary indicates that considerable progress has already been made in the control of the chief cause of death in the United States.

The problem of the extension of longevity by the control of chronic illness is twofold. The first is concerned with controlling the agents of disease and influencing host resistance. These preventive methods have been discussed in relation to syphilis and rheumatic fever.

The second aspect of control is concerned with the care that may be given individuals who already have chronic illnesses. We have discussed some of the special measures which are utilized to modify favorably the course of certain illnesses. It should be emphasized that the best results from most of these forms of treatment depend upon *early and accurate diagnosis.* The importance of frequent physical examinations to facilitate early diagnosis cannot be overemphasized. The results of special treatments now available to the chronically ill would be vitiated unless early diagnosis were established in such conditions as *pernicious anemia, pulmonary tuberculosis, pellagra, syphilis,* certain forms of *congenital heart disease,* and *cirrhosis of the liver.*

The basic principle in the care of the patient with long-term illness is that he should be treated with the same fidelity and dignity usually accorded the patient with acute illness. Only within recent years has it become possible to exact this attitude. Hospital facilities for the chronically ill were inadequate because the community conscience had not been sufficiently developed to insist upon satisfactory care of the long-term patient. The chronically ill were housed in dilapidated, ancient buildings. Medical and ancillary assistance was unsatisfactory.

In the last twenty years a happy change has taken place, particularly in New York City, under the wise leadership of Mayors LaGuardia and O'Dwyer, and Commissioners Goldwater, Rappleye, Bernecker, and Kogel. Hospital authorities have recognized that the long-term patient is more concerned with his environment than a patient acutely ill, who may spend only one or two weeks in the institution. Efforts have been made to plan a hospital to give patients a reasonable degree of privacy. Individual care by nursing and social service groups has been offered. Opportunities for recreation and rehabilitation have been emphasized. It is likely that the patient with chronic illness will be given the best care if the chronic disease pavilion is part of a general hospital organization. In this way the integration of the diagnostic and therapeutic facilities of the acute and chronic services will prevent improper care of the long-term patient. Furthermore, the quality of medical care will be improved if the hospital for chronic diseases is affiliated with a medical college. The addition of a research unit serves to attract medical workers of high quality. This is reflected in an improvement in the over-all care of the patient.

There is reason to feel proud of the progress made in the community and in the clinic with respect to the improved care of the patient with chronic illness. The medical student in 1910 was taught that there were no significant measures to control favorably the course of such diseases as we have already described. Today there exist methods for complete or partial control of at least 46 such diseases, if diagnosis and treatment are started before irreversible changes have taken place. The medical student today learns that we have no means to alter significantly the course of a number of diseases such as arteriosclerosis. It is reasonable to expect that effective methods for the control of some of these diseases will be presented to the medical student of 1975, if medical research continues at its present pace. The brief references I have made to the effectiveness of cortisone and ACTH point out certain immediate directions. These substances give promise of favorably influencing such a wide variety of chronic diseases as rheumatic fever, rheumatoid arthritis, gout, periarteritis nodosa, lupus erythematosus, asthma, eczema, hay fever, and ulcerative colitis. In the course of these and related studies, information may be turned up which might give us further clues to the mechanisms operating in the aging process in man.

May I conclude by referring to a comment made by Dr. Dochez upon his acceptance of the Kober medal from the Association of American Physicians. He remarked that the recent rapid parade of medical discoveries was startling. "In the *past*," he added, "the public had expected the physician to achieve miracles; now he is performing them."

REFERENCES

Dublin, L. I., and Others. Length of Life. Rev. ed. New York, 1949.

Cowdry, E. V., ed. Problems of Ageing. 2d ed. Baltimore, 1943.

Stieglitz, E. J., ed. Geriatric Medicine. 2d ed. Philadelphia, 1948.

Rolleston, Sir Humphry. Aspects of Age, Life and Disease. New York, 1929.

Thomson, A. P. "Problems of Ageing and Chronic Sickness,

I," *British Med. J.*, July 30, 1949, pp. 243–250; *"II," ibid.*, August 6, 1949, pp. 300–305.

McCay, C. M. "Effect of Restricted Feeding upon Aging and Chronic Diseases in Rats and Dogs." *Am. J. Pub. Health,* Vol. 37, No. 5 (1947).

Rorty, James. "The Thin Rats Bury the Fat Rats." *Harper's Magazine,* May, 1949.

Stieglitz, E. J. "On Being Old Too Young." In *Perspectives in Medicine,* New York, 1948.

Seegal, David. "On Longevity and the Control of Chronic Disease." In *The Social and Biological Challenge of Our Aging Population,* New York, 1950.

Seegal, David, Henry Colcher, Richard B. Duane, Jr., and Arthur R. Wertheim. "Progress in the Control of Chronic Illness." *Hygeia,* February, 1949.

Shaw, Bernard. Back to Methuselah. New York, 1947.

FRONTIERS IN GENETICS

By Laurence H. Snyder, Sc.D.

AS THE SCIENCE of genetics approaches its first half-century mark, it is well to pause and take stock of its present position. Although speculations on problems of heredity go far back into human history, and although Mendel's pioneer researches were carried out about one hundred years ago, genetics as a science dates only from the beginning of the twentieth century. Isolated at first, and looked on with suspicion even by its parental realms of botany and zoology, it has grown and developed until now its frontiers reach in a broad sweep completely encircling it, touching and even merging with those of many older fields of endeavor.

Always an integral part of biology, one of the frontiers of genetics has become completely identified with biology's major frontier, evolution. Genetics furnishes the modern basis for the understanding of this most important subject which, after all, is the very heart of biology.

The frontiers of genetics sweep across the broad area of agriculture, where geneticists are busily engaged in the development of new and improved varieties of livestock, pets, and cultivated plants. It is not too much to say that practically every crop variety grown in this country has been developed by geneticists and plant breeders. To cite just one example of their work, hybrid corn is worth more than a billion dollars annually to agricultural economy.

The physiology of growth and development is an active portion of the genetic front, pushing deep into the fundamental problems of this field. One sector of this area is opening up a whole new break-through into chemistry, making possible the elucidation of specific processes of metabolism. Microorganisms furnish excellent tools for such research, so that this sector includes close contact with the fields of bacteriology, virology, and similar disciplines.

Physics has furnished us with the powerful weapon of radiation, and in return genetics has provided important new material for implementing its use, so that a merging of physical and genetic frontiers is rapidly being accomplished.

Genetics very early made its peace with mathematics, and, while drawing extensively upon this realm for sustenance, has been able to repay its debt handsomely in the form of new mathematical developments, particularly in biometry. This mutual participation continues unabated.

Psychology and education, fields which long resisted attempts of genetics to form liaisons, are now extending at least tentative offers of friendship. It is reasonable to hope that common frontiers will soon develop in the areas of behavior, learning, and personality.

Population studies are rapidly moving from a demographic to a genetic attack, and population genetics is at present a most active front, developing its own unique principles and laws. Closely allied to this field is anthropology, which in recent years has become a firm ally of genetics, with its most important new frontiers inextricably bound up with those of human heredity.

Through its increasing ability to specify individuality and identify individuals, and to interpret the sometimes-confused parent-child relationship, genetics has invaded the field of law, and has some advancing fronts in common with this field.

Finally, a very close rapprochement has been achieved with medicine, and the union has resulted in the development of a recent new frontier, medical genetics. Progress is very active in this area of human health and well-being. Practical advances are appearing along such lines as the detection of genetic carriers of disease, the earlier diagnosis of illnesses and anomalies, the instituting of preventive measures, and the furnishing of information to families, all on genetic grounds. All the frontiers of genetics are coordinated and working smoothly together, however, and it is not alone the study of man in health and disease that is making possible the advances in medical genetics. Just as a person needs a variety of nutritional foods for physical health and, in addition, a varied diet of intellectual foods for mental health, so a science or a branch of a science needs sustenance from many different sources. With a viewpoint such as this, it is not surprising to find, for example, that one of the most promising leads on the cause of cancer is coming from basic genetic research on the one-celled protozoan, *Paramecium,* or that some of the more valuable advances in the understanding of the metabolic disorders in man are developing under the impetus of fundamental genetic studies on the mold, *Neurospora.*

Thus the frontiers of genetics are many and varied. In the continuing battle against the forces of the unknown, genetics is moving ahead on all these fronts. In any extended battle, however, it is inevitable that there will be at any given time areas of especial activity. I shall try to pick a few of the more crucial or significant salients of the moment.

One of the most active sectors in the advancing frontiers of genetics at the present time is that involved with the problem of how genes act in the production of finished characters. The advance guard of this sector has reached its present position as a result of a connected series of events over the past few years. The opening gun was fired by Muller, who proved by means of cleverly designed experiments that it was possible to greatly increase the natural mutation rate through the use of X-rays. The order of events from that point to the present has been somewhat as follows.

The artificial production of mutations at a greatly accelerated rate has made possible the study of the genetics of microorganisms such as bacteria, molds, and yeasts. This in turn has made available a more precise tool for studying the individual chemical steps in the metabolism of living systems. The sharpened attack thus directed at biochemical reactions has opened an avenue into the hitherto impregnable redoubt of specific gene action.

To understand the present position of the front lines and the activities going on there, some of the antecedent events should be reviewed in detail. Following Muller's discovery that X-rays could induce mutations in *Drosophila,* this principle was extended to many other organisms, both animal and plant, and to other forms of high-energy radiation. Radium rays, ultraviolet radiation, infrared rays and neutrons have also been found to induce mutations and chromosomal aberrations in a wide variety of organisms.

One cause of mutations and chromosome breaks is ionizing radiation. Ionizing radiation is that which in its passage through matter ejects electrons from the atoms through which it passes, thus leaving the atom positively charged. The atom thus affected is called an ion. The density of the ionization seems to determine the type of genetic effect. Thus, X-rays produce more mutations than they do chromosomal breaks, since ionization is not dense along the path of a fast electron, although it does become denser in the tail of the path as the electron slows down.

Ionization is dense, however, along neutron paths, and this density results in a greater proportion of chromosomal breaks than of mutations following bombardment with neutrons.

Ionizing radiations include α, β and γ radiations of radioactive substances, and X-rays, protons, and neutrons. They do not include ultraviolet light. Yet ultraviolet can cause the production of mutations. It apparently does this by excitation, which is still another way of dissipating energy in tissue and thus bringing about genetic change. Excitation is the raising of an electron in a molecule or atom to a state of higher energy. X-rays and other ionizing radiations also dissipate energy in tissues by excitation, but in general this is far less efficient in producing mutations and aberrations than is ionization.

It should be mentioned in passing that no genetic effects have thus far been demonstrable as a result of other physical agents such as electricity, electrostatic radiation, supersonic radiations, and high frequency alternating potentials.

Certain chemicals have very recently been found, however, to accelerate the mutation rate. For many years geneticists had attempted to produce mutations as a result of chemical treatment, using compounds of copper, lead, iodine, ammonia, and many other substances, to no avail. During the Second World War, however, Dr. J. M. Robson of England was involved in the study of war gasses. In the course of this study he noticed that burns from mustard gas were in many ways similar to burns from X-rays. For example, the gas burns healed with difficulty, tended to break down again after healing, and showed evidence of decreased cell division.

These facts caused him to speculate that mustard gas might be effective, in the same way that X-rays were known to be, in producing mutations. Auerbach accepted this challenge, and found that treatment of the fruit fly, *Drosophila,* with mustard gas greatly increased the mutation rate.

Other investigators have been able to increase the mutation rates in such widely separated forms as mice, plants, and bacteria, using various chemicals. The usual method of treatment is to keep the experimental organisms in an atmosphere containing a fine mist, or aerosol, of a solution of the chemical, although in some experiments the solution is injected directly into the body.

Among the effective chemicals are the sulfur mustards, the nitrogen mustards, phenol, ethyl urathane, and allyl isothiocyanate; also a number of cancer-producing substances such as methylcolanthrene, benzpyrene, and dibenzanthracine. Tests of many chemicals have disclosed others which, although penetrating, toxic, or productive of blisters, are apparently ineffective in producing mutations. Among those tested with negative results are pyrene, chloracetone, picric acid, and Lewisite.

At first thought it would not seem that chemicals and radiations had anything in common, but the suggestion has been made that those chemical agents which increase the mutation rate have a distribution of electrons such that they can transfer energy to individual genes in the chromosomes. Thus the mode of action of the effective chemicals would be, after all, similar to that of radiations.

Both chemical mutagens and radiations act in an unspecific, random way on chromosomes and genes. It has never been possible to predict what particular mutation or aberration will result from any given treatment. It is not at all beyond the bounds of possibility, however, that directed mutations will some day be produced at will.

The mutation rate resulting from X-ray irradiation is linearly proportionate to the dosage: the greater the dosage, the greater the frequency of mutation, within the limits of fertility and viability. The mutation rate is independent of the wave length. Moreover, it does not matter whether a given dosage is applied all at one time or in small fractions at different times. In contrast, the rate of chromosome breakage is more nearly proportionate to the square of the dosage, and diminishes when a given dosage is spread over a longer time.

Radiation dosages are usually expressed in Roentgen units (r). One r of X-radiation or gamma radiation will result in ionization in tissues to an average extent of 1.6 ion-pairs per cubic micron, or about one and a half trillion ion-pairs per gram of tissue.

The question logically arises as to the effects on human mutation of exposure to radiation. First of all it must be remembered that in all living organisms there is a spontaneous mutation rate observable. Extensive investigations place this spontaneous rate at between 1 in 100,000 and 1 in 1,000,000 per gene per generation. These figures seem to hold regardless of the length of the generation, be it ten days in *Drosophila* or twenty-five years in man. The mutation rate for man is apparently nearer the higher rate, being, for some half dozen genes carefully studied, between 1 and 4 per 100,000.

Natural irradiation, such as cosmic rays and local gamma radiation, total only about 0.1 r per year, or less than 3 r from birth to average child-bearing age. Inasmuch as 1 r will result on the average in an induced mutation rate of only 1 per 33,000,000, it is apparent that natural irradiation is not nearly sufficient to account for the natural spontaneous mutation rate. This rate must largely result from other causes, such as the natural random inter- and intramolecular motions.

What, then, will exposure to irradiation do to people? In a masterly analysis, Evans has thoroughly investigated the possibilities. Those persons whose daily work is with radioactive substances and radiations are by agreement limited to a whole-body dosage of 0.1 r per working day. In practice, due to careful protective measures, workers will seldom actually receive that much. At most this would total 250 r in a ten-year working period before the age of parenthood.

On the average, radiation workers will receive only about 20 r during their working lives prior to the production of children. Even if an individual received the entire maximum allowable dosage of 250 r, however, this would add only about the equivalent of the natural mutation occurrence. Since every person undoubtedly carries an accumulation of mutated genes far greater than the number which have mutated in his own generation, 250 r of irradiation would add only one or two mutations to every hundred spontaneously occurring mutations already accumulated in his cells.

From these facts Evans concludes that no detectable increase in hereditary abnormalities is likely to result, even after many generations, if a small fraction of the population receives daily radiation doses up to 0.1 r per day.

There would be danger, of course, if persons exposed to irradiation should be careless, and allow their testes or ovaries to receive excessive dosages. The greatest of caution should be observed by those concerned in any way with active X-ray, fluoroscopic, and similar equipment, since larger doses than the minimal allowable may certainly be expected to result in genetic change.

Thus in recent years it has been amply demonstrated that radiation and certain chemicals in appropriate dosages can greatly accelerate the natural mutation rate. This means that geneticists need no longer wait for mutations to happen at the exceedingly slow natural rate, but that mutations may be produced in relatively large numbers for study and analysis, by artificial means. This principle has been used freely, particularly in agriculture, and mutations have been produced in many crop plants and in a few experimental animals.

The significant break-through in this line of advance came, however, when Beadle and Tatum realized that the practicability of artificially inducing mutations made it possible to attempt the large-scale study of the genetics of microorganisms. It was clear that the vital chemical reactions of metabolism took place within cells, and that genes might in some way direct or control these reactions. It would therefore be profitable to work with an organism which could be studied both biochemically and genetically.

Lindegren, Dodge, and others had already demonstrated the advantages possessed by yeasts and molds in genetic analysis. Beadle and Tatum saw that by inducing large numbers of mutations in such organisms, their peculiarly favorable genetic potentialities might be used to advantage in biochemical studies. Such studies might in turn lead to an approach to the solution of the problem of how genes act in the production of specific characteristics. These hopes have been abundantly justified in recent years.

In the early days of the study of genetics, the geneticist was content to establish the correlation between the gene in the chromosome and the characteristic in the individual, without raising much question as to the chain of events which connected the two. The attitude was very much like that of the traveler who boards the Miami train in New York, confident that he will step out at the Miami station, but actually knowing very little about the physicochemical principles of the Diesel engine or the intracacies of the switching and signaling systems that will get him there.

Today, however, the question of genic action in the development of finished characters is uppermost in the minds of geneticists, and biochemical genetics is leading the attack on this front.

The bread mold, *Neurospora,* is of especial importance for biochemical genetic studies because of a number of facts. First, the larger part of its life cycle, as in other lower plants, consists of a structure in which the cells are haploid, that is, they contain but one of each pair of chromosomes, and thus one of each gene. In one sense, all the cells of the mold correspond to the gametes of an animal. Thus any gene may produce its effect in the cells of the mold: there is no complication of dominance or recessiveness; and the commonly observed Mendelian ratio will be one to one.

Second, there is a diploid generation in the life cycle of the mold, in which the chromosomes and genes are in pairs, but this is limited to a single cell-generation. Its occurrence, however, makes it possible to cross two haploid strains, recombine the genes, and map the chromosomes.

Third, and extremely important, the bread mold, unlike man, is capable of synthesizing all the purines, pyramidines, and amino acids which it needs for its development, and all the "vitamins" but one. In other words, the mold can live and grow on a basic medium containing merely a source of energy and carbon; a suitable source of nitrogen, such as ammonium salts; a source of inorganic elements such as salts supplying calcium, phosphate, sulfur, potassium and iron; and the one vitamin which the mold can not make, namely biotin, one of the B-vitamins. From this basic medium *Neurospora* can synthesize at least 20 amino acids, many vitamins, purines, pyramidines, and nucleic acids, and other substances which go to make up the mold.

Beadle and his colleagues knew that irradiation caused mutations, and that the mutated genes were usually inactive, or at least less active, in carrying out the particular functions which they formerly controlled. They reasoned that irradiation of *Neurospora* spores might be expected to inactivate genes which controlled the metabolism of one or another of the various substances built up by the mold from the basic medium. If this occurred, it should be possible to deduce, from the change thus brought about, the role of the unmutated, normal gene.

Accordingly, asexual spores of *Neurospora* were irradiated, and then added to a normal culture of the opposite sex, thus achieving a cross. The sexual spores resulting from the cross were grown individually on complete media containing all the substances necessary for growth and functioning of the mold. This, of course, was to insure that the mutations, if any, would be preserved. After obtaining a profuse vegetative growth, part of each culture was transferred to the basic medium. If it grew there, no mutation interfering with the production of essential substances had occurred. If it did not grow on the minimal medium, a mutation had apparently taken place preventing the synthesis of some vitamin, amino acid, or other necessary building block.

About one or two cultures out of every hundred irradiated showed inability to grow on the minimal medium. It was then necessary to discover what particular substance was no longer being synthesized by the mold. A culture was therefore tried on a minimal medium to which all the known vitamins had been added, and another on a minimal medium to which all the amino acids had been added.

If the culture then grew in the presence of vitamins but not in the presence of amino acids, it was evidence that this strain had lost the ability to produce some one of the vitamins which it formerly could produce. If it grew in the presence of the amino acids but not of the vitamins, it had lost the power to synthesize some amino acid. If perchance it grew on neither culture, it had lost the power to synthesize some necessary substance other than the known vitamins or amino acids.

Suppose a particular treated strain will grow on minimal medium supplemented with vitamins, but not on a supplement of amino acids. It is then necessary to determine just which vitamin is no longer synthesized. The strain is then tried on a series of minimal media, each supplemented with one vitamin, such as riboflavin, niacin, thiamin, and so on. In this way the strain is found to be incapable of synthesizing a particular specific substance.

Next it must be determined whether or not the change is connected with a gene. This is done by crossing the new strain with an opposite-sexed untreated strain. If the two strains differ by a single gene mutation, half of the resulting spores will give rise to the original kind of mold, and half to the new kind.

Tests of hundreds of thousands of spores have revealed many mutations as a result of irradiation, each mutation making the mold incapable of synthesizing a particular substance. For example, various mutated strains can not make, respectively, vitamins B_1, B_2, B_6, niacin, choline, inositol, pantothenic acid or *p*- aminobenzoic acid. Other strains can no longer synthesize one or another of the amino acids phenylalanine, leucine, valine, isoleucine, arginine, proline, lysine, tryptophane, threonine, ornithine, citrulline, and methionine. Still others cannot build specific purines or pyrimidines, substances which go to make up nucleic acids, the principle components of chromosomes, and probably of genes.

At this point the union of genetics and biochemistry becomes apparent. Genetic research discloses the fact that each failure in synthesis is the result of a single gene mutation. Biochemical research makes it clear that each failure is the result of a lack of a specific enzyme. In general, each step in the chemical reactions occurring in the cells of living organisms takes place under the influence of a specific enzyme, and in the absence of the enzyme either will not take place or will proceed at such a slow rate as not to be very effective.

Furthermore we know, due to the work of Sumner and those who followed him, that all the enzymes that have been adequately purified and analyzed are proteins. We also know, as a result of the researches of Mirsky and his colleagues, that genes consist of, or at least contain, proteins.

It is not difficult, then, to accept Beadle's suggestion that the genes serve as permanent models in the images of which enzyme proteins are constructed. Enzymes are very specific, and it seems highly probable that each enzyme is referable to a single gene. In other words, the genes appear to direct the production of specific enzyme proteins, and these in turn control specific chemical reactions.

On this hypothesis a mutation, either natural or induced, is thought of as being an alteration in the chemical arrangement of the protein molecule. The mutated gene, in its reproduction, duplicates itself in its altered form just as faithfully as it previously copied its original form. This is one of the foundation stones of evolution. Furthermore, the protein molecule after mutation is usually inactive, or at least less active, in catalyzing the particular reaction which it formerly brought about.

Practical applications of this knowledge have been many. Such forms as *Neurospora* can be used in bioassays, for determining qualitatively and quantitatively the presence of individual vitamins, amino acids, and other substances. Moreover, the steps in the syntheses of such substances can be worked out, and the precursors identified. In this way we have learned, for example, the steps leading from ornithine through citrulline to arginine, and those proceeding from anthranilic acid to indole, followed by condensation with serine, resulting in tryptophane. Research along similar lines is in active progress at the present time, involving many biosynthetic processes, and making use of other organisms such as yeasts and bacteria.

Examples of the production of traits through the genic control of biochemical reactions are not lacking in man. A recently discovered disease is known as phenylketonuria. Those who suffer from this disease are mentally deficient, frequently being institutionalized, and appear like other idiots and imbeciles in every way but one. Analysis of the urine of such individuals reveals that they excrete about a gram per day of an abnormal metabolite, phenylpyruvic acid. This substance is the keto-acid analogue of phenylalanine, one of the indispensable amino acids in our diet.

Phenylalanine is handled by the cells in various ways. Some of it goes to make up our body proteins. Some of it, however, is oxidized to phenylpyruvic acid by replacing its amino group by an oxygen atom. Normally we then degrade phenylpyruvic acid by successive steps through parahydroxyphenylpyruvic acid, 2, 5- dihydroxyphenylpyruvic acid, homogentisic acid and aceto-acetic acid to carbon dioxide and water. Each of these steps requires the presence of a specific enzyme. All these enzymes are produced by normal individuals.

Affected individuals, however, cannot convert phenylpyruvic acid to parahydroxyphenylpyruvic acid. Lacking the requisite enzyme, the former substance is piled up and finally excreted in the urine. The accumulation in some way affects normal mental processes, and the result is mental deficiency. Careful genetic studies by Folling and Penrose have made it clear that phenylketonuria is the result of a single autosomal recessive gene substitution.

Hence it appears that the normal allele of this gene brings about the production of the enzyme necessary to convert phenylpyruvic acid to the parahydroxy form, while the mutated gene fails to produce this enzyme.

Other human diseases seem to be brought about in a similar manner. If the conversion of phenylpyruvic acid to the parahydroxy form is made, the next step in the process may fail to occur, in which case parahydroxyphenylpyruvic acid is accumulated, and the individual has tyrosinosis. If this step is carried out, another mutant gene, if present, will result in the absence of the enzyme necessary to degrade homogentisic acid to aceto-acetic acid. The accumulation and excretion of homogentisic acid results in the abnormal condition known as alcaptonuria.

While some of the original phenylalanine is being built into proteins, and some is being degraded through the keto-acid chain just described, still other amounts of it are metabolized by a different series of oxidations through parahydroxyphenylalanine, the 3, 4-dihydroxy form, and a series of other forms, ending up with melanin, the pigment of our skin, eyes, and hair. Normally pigmented persons produce all the enzymes necessary to make each of these steps, but an occasional individual inherits in homozygous form a mutant gene which fails to produce the enzyme necessary to break down the 3, 4-dihydroxyphenylalanine. Melanin is not produced, and the individual is an albino.

Not only is amino acid metabolism subject to breaks in the chain of reactions, but lipid and carbohydrate metabolism are also interfered with by lack of appropriate enzymes. Carbohydrate metabolism is being extensively studied with yeasts by Lindegren and others. Again, recent research is providing examples in man.

Normal individuals carry glycogen through glucose -1- phosphate and glucose -6- phosphate to glucose and H_3PO_4.

Those having Von Gierke's disease, however, fail to produce the enzyme phosphorylase and so do not degrade glycogen, which thus piles up in the liver, heart, kidneys, and other organs during infancy, causing characteristic symptoms. Other derangements of carbohydrate metabolism, such as diabetes, pentosuria, and fructosuria might be discussed at some length were space available.

Turning to lipid metabolism, an interesting human example is Tay-Sach's disease, in which the affected infant becomes blind, paralyzed, and mentally deficient; and invariably dies within a short time. Here the oxidation of the lipid sphyngomyelin, which takes place in normal individuals, fails to occur. Many other examples, such as failure to metabolize kerasin in Gaucher's disease, or cholesterol in xanthomatosis, could be cited.

Each of the human diseases listed above apparently results from the lack of a specific enzyme, and each seems to be genetically the result of a single mutated gene substitution. Medical genetics thus provides additional evidence for the growing belief in a one-to-one correspondence between gene and enzyme. It is of interest in this connection that the researches of Lea indicate that on the basis of ionization effects, genes appear to have diameters of 4 to 8 millimicrons, and molecular weights of from 50,000 to 500,000. These values fall within the size and weight ranges of enzymes.

The one-to-one relationship between gene and enzyme probably also applies to other protein products of the gene. I shall discuss this later on in connection with antigens. It should be pointed out here, however, that there are inherent in biochemical genetics implications for the understanding not only of particular diseases and anomalies, but also of the organism as a whole. It is not too much to hope that the day will arrive when the genetic basis for the complete metabolic processes of man may be built into a single mosaic. Since several of the inherited metabolic derangements, such as Tay-Sach's disease, epilepsy, and phenylketonuria, involve severe mental defects, it is also within the range of possibility that the study of biochemical genetics will make it possible to specify the entire nervous and mental make-up of an individual in terms of measurable inherited metabolic activities. These things are among the shining goals of the medical geneticist.

It is relatively easy to understand how one gene, acting through an enzyme, can result in a restricted effect, such as eye color, but more difficult to comprehend at first glance a wide-spread fundamental effect such as the complete syndrome of Tay-Sach's disease. Presumably it is partly, at least, a matter of timing: of the critical period of development at which the gene acts.

To return to our analogy of the train, let us suppose that you have boarded a train in New York. Just outside the Pennsylvania station is a switch. If it is thrown one way, you will end up somewhere in the south, possibly Miami; whereas if it is thrown the other way you will end up in the west, perhaps Chicago. A simple switch acting at an early stage of your journey can make a tremendous difference in the outcome.

Assume now that the switch has been thrown so as to send you south. It is now determined that you will not proceed west, but there is yet the opportunity of ending up at, let us say, either Miami or New Orleans. The positions of various switches along the route will determine this, but at least you will end up in the south as opposed to the west.

Let us assume, however, that you finally approach Miami. Just outside the Miami station is another switch, similar in its intrinsic action to the others. But whether this switch is thrown one way or the other will make only the specific and relatively slight difference as to whether you arrive on Track 1 or Track 2 of the Miami terminal.

Thus an early effective gene such as the recessive determiner for Tay-Sach's disease, which fails to produce the enzyme necessary for the oxidation of the lipid sphyngomyelin, may result in profound physical and mental disturbances. On the other hand, the recessive gene which fails to form the enzyme necessary for the production of pigment in the iris, acting very specifically and at a relatively late point in the development of the eye, may make only the difference between being brown eyed or blue eyed.

But I have taken perhaps an undue portion of my time on biochemical genetics, important as this frontier is. Let us turn to other active sectors, and consider first the recent incursions into the area of extranuclear determiners of heredity.

One of the major conclusions of genetic research during the past half-century has been that traits are determined, in so far as genetic differences provide the effective variables, by mutable, self-duplicating genes located at specific points in the chromosomes. Now, however, an entirely new front is opening up, indicating that some genetic variability may be the result of similar mutable, self-duplicating units, located not in the chromosomes, but in the cytoplasm. One type of such cytoplasmic transmission, plastid inheritance in plants, has long been known, but it was until recently considered an isolated and unique example.

Chloroplasts are relatively large cytoplasmic bodies occurring in the cells of green plants. They contain chlorophyll, the green coloring matter which is involved in the process of photosynthesis. They are self-perpetuating bodies which are distributed more or less at random to the two daughter cells when a plant cell divides. Mutations can occur in plastids, and one such mutation makes the plastid defective in that it no longer synthesizes chlorophyll. Cytoplasm containing such defective plastids is devoid of chlorophyll, and appears white.

In the leaves of certain strains of four-o'clocks, for example, colorless plastids may occur among the green ones. Such leaves are variegated green and white. Sometimes a whole branch is white, containing only defective plastids in its cytoplasm. Again, a whole branch may be green, containing only normal plastids.

When flowers on an all-white branch are pollinated with pollen from a green branch, the resulting offspring are white. Conversely, when flowers on a green branch are pollinated with pollen from a white branch, the resulting plants are all green. In other words, the offspring resemble only the mother in regard to leaf and stem color. Since the plastids are cytoplasmic structures, and ordinarily no cytoplasm is brought in by the sperm at fertilization, this type of transmission appears to be extranuclear, nonchromosomal, and non-Mendelian in nature.

Other examples of cytoplasmic inheritance have recently been brought to light, some of them with far-reaching implications for biological theory and even for medical practice. Among these examples are structural characters in mosses, sterility in various plants, reciprocal differences in size and shape of various parts in the evening primrose, pathogenicity in rusts, color in wasps, sensitivity to carbon dioxide in *Drosophila,* and a number of characters in *Paramecium.*

The researches of Sonneborn and his collaborators with *Paramecium* are of especial importance, and a brief outline of some of them will be of value in understanding the implications of this type of work. Although many of the characters of this unicellular organism are controlled by genes carried in the chromosomes in the nucleus, other characters are apparently cytoplasmically determined. Sonneborn calls the cytoplasmic determiners plasmagenes. There are many different kinds of plasmagenes in *Paramecium,* each self-reproducing and capable of mutation. Plasmagenes depend for their maintenance and reproduction on nuclear genes, however, and are therefore not completely autonomous. A brief description of one of these plasmagenes and its action will serve to illustrate the general developments in this very new frontier.

Genes are traditionally named with Roman letters: *a, b, c,* and so on. The convention has arisen of naming plasmagenes with Greek letters: alpha, beta, gamma, and so forth. The plasmagene most thoroughly studied in *Paramecium* is one called kappa. When it is present in the cytoplasm in sufficient concentration it results in the production of an extracellular antibiotic agent called paramecin. This substance will kill paramecia of certain strains known as "sensitives," although it does not affect those strains which produce it, known as "killers."

Kappa can be maintained in an individual and its progeny only when the dominant gene *K* is present in the nucleus. Thus individuals of genotypes *KK* and *Kk* may be killers; those of genotype *kk* are always sensitives. However, the mere presence of gene *K* in the nucleus does not insure the presence of kappa. Kappa must come from preexisting kappa by its own reproduction.

The modes of reproduction of *Paramecium* are varied and complicated, and it is not possible to go into them in detail here. Suffice it to say that by proper manipulation it is possible to replace gene *K* by its allele *k* in a killer animal. When this is done, the animal gradually loses its kappa and becomes sensitive. If now the original *K* is brought back into the cell by suitable crossing, it cannot recreate kappa, and the individual will remain sensitive.

A killer individual must, then, contain both the gene *K* and a suitable concentration of kappa. The concentration necessary to make an individual a killer is several hundred kappa particles. The reproduction of plasmagenes is not necessarily correlated with the rate of cell division, so that by suitable manipulation of the cultural conditions it is possible to bring the concentration of kappa to any desired level and maintain it there. When a killer animal with several hundred kappa plasmagenes is so manipulated as to reduce its supply of kappa, it first stops producing paramecin, although remaining resistant; then becomes sensitive, even though it retains the gene *K*.

Now these facts show a remarkable similarity to a series of discoveries in regard to cancer. In mice, for example, there are strains in which practically every animal develops mammary cancer; others in which almost no animal ever does. Crosses between these strains indicated that the inheritance of the tumors was largely maternal, hence cytoplasmic, or at least extrachromosomal.

Further studies by Bittner indicated that the transmission was largely on the basis of some substance, probably a virus, in the mother's milk.

Recent research by Heston and his colleagues indicates a strong resemblance between the milk agent in mice and kappa in *Paramecium.* For example, the maintenance of the milk agent is dependent upon certain genes in mice just as that of kappa is dependent upon the gene *K* in *Paramecium.* Again, just as certain sensitive strains of the protozoan may have *K* but lack kappa, so certain noncancerous strains of mice have the requisite genes but lack the milk agent. In addition, the transfer of the milk agent through milk from foster mothers to mice having the cancer genes, but lacking the agent, will result in these animals maintaining the milk agent and transmitting it, just as was done with kappa by adding it to strains lacking it but having gene *K*. Finally, Heston and his colleagues showed that it was possible to maintain the milk factor at low concentration with no resulting cancer, just as Sonneborn had been able to do with kappa and the resulting lack of production of the antibiotic paramecin.

The above facts raise the question as to the fundamental differences, if any, between plasmagenes and viruses. Both are located outside the chromosomes; both are self-duplicating, but only in the requisite genotype; both are mutable and reproduce the mutated form; both result in definite characters. If they differ at all, it would appear to be in the conceptions that plasmagenes are transmitted by a type of heredity and are normal cell constituents, while viruses are transmitted by infection and are abnormal, pathogenic cell dwellers. Darlington, Haddow, Sonneborn, and others have speculated on these facts. It has been pointed out that what is a virus in one species or variety may be a plasmagene in another, in the same way that thiamine is a vitamin for man but is normally synthesized by *Neurospora,* and is thus not a vitamin for the mold.

For example, a plasmagene in one variety of potato acts as a pathogenic virus when transferred to another variety. Other examples both in plants and in animals are known. It may be, then, as Darlington suggests, that a virus is merely a plasmagene in the wrong host.

There has been formulated, on the basis of facts such as these, the plasmagene theory of cancer. This theory involves the production of cancer by somatic mutations of plasmagenes, resulting in the release of the ordinary inhibitions regulating cell growth and division. The various known carcinogenic agents would, on this theory, either make the cells more receptive to foreign plasmagenes (viruses) or cause mutations of native plasmagenes. As was pointed out in an earlier section of this review, chemical carcinogens are known to produce mutations.

On the plasmagene theory of cancer the lag between the application of the carcinogen and the appearance of the cancer would be readily explained. When a few particles of kappa are introduced into a *Paramecium* lacking kappa but having *K*, the kappa increases gradually under proper conditions. When it reaches the level of several hundred particles, the cell becomes a killer instead of being sensitive. It may very well be in cancer that the mutated plasmagene must slowly increase to the critical cellular concentration requisite for cancer manifestation.

The older theory of the gene clearly requires modification. There is no reason now to doubt the existence of cytoplasmic units: mutable, self-duplicating, and capable of controlling the development of characters, but in turn controlled by nuclear genes. Specific, localizable, Mendelizing, chromosomal genes and specific cytoplasmic plasmagenes, some of which are localizable in visible cytoplasmic structures, must both be taken into account in formulating a modern theory of the gene. Such a theory may give the clues to many enigmas of biology.

Classical genetic experiments have long been performed under controlled conditions in the laboratory or field plot. Analytical methods for dealing with the results of such experiments have been prepared by mathematical geneticists. Especially in regard to the problems of evolution have the mathematicians made progress. Wright, Haldane, Fisher, and others have substituted exact quantitative considerations for the speculative approach, even to encompassing the whole evolutionary process within a single mathematical framework. As a matter of fact, the theoretical considerations have tended to outstrip the empirical investigations of evolutionary processes.

Recently, however, the front line of attack on evolution in the field has shown signs of increasing activity. Although the classical methods of genetics continue to be of the highest value, observers are turning more and more to what Professor Dunn has called "that ultimate laboratory, free nature itself." Careful year-round analyses of the frequencies of various genes and chromosomal arrangements have been made in wild populations of flies, beetles, hamsters, foxes, roses, grasses, and many other organisms. Dobzhansky, Spencer, Clausen, Stebbins, Gershenson, Timmofeeff-Ressovsky, Dubinin and many others are engaged in such studies. As a result it is proving perfectly feasible actually to observe evolutionary processes in action. Future discussions of natural selection, adaptive systems, isolation barriers, species reservoirs of potential adaptive variability, and other evolutionary mechanisms need no longer be carried on from the purely speculative angle. Empirical data are rapidly being accumulated, and the near future should bring into sharp focus many hitherto blurred considerations of evolution.

Investigations in population genetics have not been confined to wild animals and plants, but have been made with increasing vigor in human material. The studies of Dahlberg, Haldane, Rife, Snyder, Wiener, Wright, and others have resulted in the formulation of a series of principles of human population genetics. Moreover, in all parts of the world data are beginning to appear on the population frequencies of various human genes.

In regard to human populations, we now utilize a number of principles which were not until recently clearly recognized. Some of these are as follows.

1. Classical Mendelian ratios are not to be expected in random samples from a free-breeding population, nor even necessarily from the pooled offspring of a series of families

where the parental mating types are outwardly alike. Classical Mendelian ratios are to be looked for only among the offspring of an individual family (if there are sufficient offspring), or among the pooled offspring of a series of families where the parental mating types are actually genetically alike. Since the genotypes of human beings are seldom capable of specification, even the best classified data will usually contain mixtures of different types of matings, and thus must not be expected to demonstrate classical Mendelian ratios.

2. In spite of the lack of observable classical ratios, predictable ratios of another sort do occur under the conditions stated above. These are *population ratios,* in contrast to Mendelian ratios. They are expressed in terms of the proportions in the population of the genes concerned, and their values vary as these proportions vary. In matings of two individuals exhibiting a dominant trait, for example, there are involved three static Mendelian ratios, namely 3/4 : 1/4, 1/2 : 1/2, and 1 : 0. In a random-mating population these are jointly expressed as one dynamic population ratio,

$$\frac{1 + 2q}{(1 + q)^2} : \frac{q^2}{(1 + q)^2},$$

where q is the proportion of the recessive gene in the population. Many similar population ratios have been derived.

3. The comparison of predicted and observed population ratios may serve as a basis for estimating the number and kind of genes responsible for a hereditary variation in a population, just as the comparison of predicted and observed Mendelian ratios may serve as a basis for estimating the number and kind of genes involved in a laboratory experiment. Formulations by Cotterman, Haldane, Hogben, Snyder, Wiener, and others are providing the requisite goodness-of-fit tests.

4. The mechanisms of segregation and recombination are such that, in a large population in which the effects of mutation and selection and in-and-out-migration are either negligible or balancing each other, the proportions of the various genes will remain constant from generation to generation. If, in addition, there is random mating in a constant environment in the population, the proportions of the gene combinations (genotypes), and thus of the traits produced by them, will likewise remain constant.

5. Changes in the frequencies of genes and traits cannot be brought about by the mere dominance or recessiveness of specific hereditary factors, popular belief to the contrary notwithstanding. Such changes can be brought about, however, by various phenomena, including mutation, selection, inbreeding, assortative mating, the restriction of matings within social or geographic isolates, migration, and, particularly in small populations, random drift of gene proportions. The rates and extents of the changes so produced are capable of exact mathematical formulation, and have been discussed in recent books by Dahlberg, Hogben, Li, and others.

6. A demonstrated correlation between the occurrence of two traits in a randomly breeding population does not necessarily indicate linkage between the genes determining these traits.

Theoretical considerations of population genetics are far in advance of empirical investigations, and we are just beginning to realize the necessity of carefully collected genetic field data on man. Fortunately physical anthropologists as well as geneticists are rapidly absorbing this viewpoint, and such data are now being accumulated. Their collection involves much more than the mere counting of the respective frequences of contrasting traits and their distribution within families, however, and must include information on the extent of the formation of isolates, the systems of mating practiced, and the extent of the use of such systems.

As genetic data on human populations accumulate, one clear fact seems to be emerging. Human populations appear to differ genetically one from the other almost entirely in the varying *proportions* of the allelic genes of the various sets of hereditary factors, and not in the *kinds* of genes they contain. Judging by the populations studied, it would appear that no large population in the world completely lacks any allele, but that one population may contain a larger or a smaller proportion of a given allele than another, and that these varying proportions constitute the major genetic differences between races. Thus the extreme positions held by those who on the one hand claim that there are no genetic differences between human races, and those who on the other hand hold that certain races are "superior" and others "inferior" require drastic modification in the light of modern advances in the genetic study of human populations.

The frontiers of population genetics merge into those of medical genetics, and both are very active at the present time. Among the advance sectors of this frontier are a series of applications of medical genetics to the practice of medicine. These include the clinical detection of the genetic carriers of disease, the instituting of therapeutic and preventive measures based on such detection, the making of genetic prognoses, the earlier and more accurate diagnosis of disease based on genetic data; and the solution of medical problems such as hemolytic disease of the newborn, and medicolegal problems such as the determination of disputed paternity, based on the inheritance of the various blood groups and types. There is room for the detailed discussion of only one or two of these applications.

Let us consider one of the most important of these advance sectors, our increasing ability to detect the genetic carriers of disease. Detectable genetic carriers are of several sorts. First there are those persons who carry a dominant gene with variable expressivity. Some of them may exhibit the complete clinical picture at the time of examination, but others may show only one or another of the preclinical, laboratory stigmata. Those showing the early signs may later develop the full-blown condition. In the meantime, preventive measures may be applied to forestall the clinical manifestations.

Examples of the foregoing application are found in a number of diseases. Gout for instance, is apparently the result of a dominant gene for hyperuricemia. When the mean uric acid level exceeds a certain value for a certain period, clinical gout develops. Meanwhile the hyperuricemia may be recognized and the carrier identified.

Hemolytic icterus, in which the clinical symptoms are jaundice and marked anemia, sometimes resulting in sudden death, is the result of a dominant gene. The early signs manifested by a person carrying the gene are certain changes in the size, shape, structure, and function of the red cells, and an enlarged spleen. Where one or another of these signs is found in the relatives of a patient with clinical manifestations, appropriate prophylactic surgery may be instituted.

Xanthoma tuberosum is the result of a dominant gene for increased blood cholesterol and cholesterol esters. This can be detected early, before the complete clinical picture develops, involving nodules and tumors of the tendons and joints. Dietary therapy may then be instituted.

Epilepsy seems to develop under the influence of a dominant gene resulting in cerebral dysrhythmia, an abnormal type of brain wave which can be demonstrated by means of a recording apparatus known as the electroencephalograph.

Some of those showing cerebral dysrhythmia proceed to clinical epilepsy. The carriers can thus be recognized by appropriate measurements, and although very little can be done at present in the way of preventive therapy, those who can transmit the condition can at least be identified.

Pernicious anemia is another disease in which carriers may be recognized. The gene or genes concerned result in a prolonged achlorhydria (absence of hydrochloric acid from the gastric juice). This may be followed by clinical pernicious anemia or hypochromic anemia. Appropriate preventive therapy may be applied to the carriers.

Other diseases possibly due to dominant genes with varying degrees of penetrance or expressivity are in process of analysis from the standpoint of detecting carriers. These include such conditions as diabetes mellitus and essential hypertension.

A second type of detectable genetic carriers of disease includes those persons heterozygous for a gene which in the homozygous state produces a clinical anomaly, but who themselves may show some minor but significant departure from the norm. Recent research has disclosed many such instances. For example, those heterozygous for the gene for thalassemia, a chronic, progressive, fatal anemia of childhood, show a mild microcytic anemia with characteristic "target cells," together with a decreased fragility in hypotonic saline solutions. Similar identification of heterozygotes is proving to be possible in such conditions as sickle cell anemia, phenylketonuria, hemophilia, one type of sex-linked microcytic anemia, afibrinogenemia, a sex-linked type of retinitis pigmentosa, and several ectodermal derangements such as keratosis, xeroderma pigmentosum, and the absence of sweat glands.

Another type of detectable carrier is being found in certain anomalies which have long been thought to be the results of dominant genes, although only the heterozygous condition was formerly known. It now appears that some of these genes, when they do occur in homozygous state, produce a new set of symptoms, usually far more severe, even lethal. Thus, for example, the relatively harmless heterozygous anomaly known as hemorrhagic telangiectasia appears in the homozygous state as a severe, fulminating lethal condition. The allergy of adults is the heterozygous form of very severe childhood allergic manifestations. The gene which in heterozygous state produces a minor brachydactyly (short fingers), results in the homozygous form in the absence of fingers and toes. Other similar instances are being brought to light.

Neel has recently summarized this valuable new line of research, and has pointed out, as have Macklin, Snyder, and others, that such detection of genetic carriers will make possible a sharpened approach to the physiology of disease and to the mode of action of the genes concerned, by providing for study a relatively large number of persons in the very early stages of the condition.

Moreover, by searching for and finding the early stigmata, slight but significant deviations from the norm, which have in the past been ignored by physician and patient alike, will take on a new and important meaning in the light of genetics, resulting in new criteria for diagnosis, earlier identification, and consequent new opportunities for prevention and therapy. Under this new viewpoint it is not too much to hope, as Macklin has so clearly pointed out, that just as diagnosis has shifted in the last half century from the autopsy to the biopsy, so with the aid of medical genetics it may be expected to move even further back to a point where the patient is not only alive, but shows only such signs of incipient disease or anomaly as have hitherto been unrecognized and untreated.

The front lines of activity in medical genetics are extremely varied, and it is not possible here to describe them all, but it would be a major oversight to leave out some consideration of the remarkable recent work of Wiener, Levine, Race, and others on the rapidly expanding series of blood groups and types. When I presented the Biggs Lecture before The New York Academy of Medicine in 1946, I listed 3,200 different blood groups in man, with the possibility in the near future of knowing 8,640 different combinations. During those three years, due to the discovery of additional new hemagglutinogens in man, the number of combinations which can result in distinct blood groups has risen to 4,147,200.

Large as this number seems, it is still small compared with the number of comparable antigenic differences which have recently been demonstrated in cattle by Irwin and his associates. By means of appropriate immune antiserums they have found in cattle forty antigens, each genetically determined, and each capable of being present or absent in any individual animal. The number of known possible "blood groups" in cattle is thus 2^{40}, which is more than a trillion. It would appear that any individual cow or bull in the country can be specifically identified by its blood group.

In man we now know at least twenty-five inherited blood antigens (hemagglutinogens), which in their various combinations are capable of forming the more than four million distinct human blood groups. Of course some of the various antigens are rare in all populations, so that certain combinations of them will be highly improbable. Nevertheless all the millions of combinations are potentially possible, and many of them exist with reasonable frequencies. It is highly unlikely, for example, that any two of my readers have the same blood group.

Each of the twenty-five known agglutinogens in man is

inherited in a simple Mendelian manner, with the result that a child never has a specific antigen unless at least one of the parents had it. This fact is, of course, the basis for the medicolegal aspects of the blood groups, since if a child does possess one of these antigens and the mother lacks it, the father must have had it. A man lacking the specific antigen involved could not, therefore, be the father of the child.

The various antigens are found in different proportions from race to race, and they follow the laws of population genetics within each ethnic group or other isolate just as they follow the laws of Mendelian genetics within families. They also exhibit varying degrees of antigenicity in man, and may or may not have natural antibodies in human individuals. Here again frontiers merge, those of genetics being at this point one with those of immunology.

The known human hemagglutinogens fall into three major categories. First there are those represented by the familiar A-B blood group antigens, long known to be important in transfusions because each agglutinogen is not only antigenic to man but is reciprocally matched by a normal antibody occurring in the serum and other body fluids of persons not having the specific antigen. At least four antigens of this sort are known.

Second, there are those represented by the M-N blood type antigens, weakly if at all antigenic to man, so that antibodies against them can be produced only by animals. Hence they are unimportant in transfusions, although of value in medicolegal cases. At least six antigens of this sort have been described and studied.

Third, there are those hemagglutinogens represented by the Rh factors which, like the second kind, have no natural antibodies in man, but which are, on occasion at least, highly antigenic to man, so that transfusion from a donor having one of these antigens to a recipient not having it may result in immunizing the recipient. The transfusion may be intentional, such as in therapy, or unintentional, such as may occur from an embryo to its mother.

At least fifteen hemagglutinogens of this third kind have been described in man in the last few years, and more will undoubtedly be found in the near future. The best known of this category is the well-publicized Rh factor, about which something should be said here, since it is certainly in the center of one of the most active genetic frontiers at the present moment.

The original Rh antigen was discovered by Landsteiner and Wiener through the injection of red blood cells from the rhesus monkey into animals, thus immunizing the animals and resulting in the production of an antibody which would agglutinate the cells of the monkey. When tried on human red cells, this antibody would agglutinate the cells of some persons and not others. Using the first two letters of rhesus, the newly discovered antigen was named "Rh." Although the first antibody against it was produced by animals, it is now known that Rh and similar antigens more recently discovered are antigenic to man, so that at present human immune serums are used as the source of antibodies for testing the occurrence of these antigens.

Two important applications have arisen from the fact that although there are no natural antibodies against Rh, it is antigenic to man. One of these applications is not genetic and involves intentional transfusion. Although the first transfusion of Rh-positive blood into an Rh-negative recipient can cause no immediate transfusion reaction because of the absence of natural antibodies, it can cause immunization, resulting in the eventual production of antibodies by the recipient. A later transfusion of Rh-positive blood might then result in a dangerous reaction. Rh-negative individuals must always be transfused with Rh-negative blood.

The second application is definitely a genetic one; it involves a severe disease of newborn infants. It was discovered by Levine and his associates that an inadvertent transfusion sometimes occurs across the placenta from an embryo to its mother. If the embryo is Rh positive and the mother Rh negative, the results will be similar to those occurring in therapeutic transfusions, that is, the mother may become immunized and stimulated to produce antibodies against Rh. The first Rh-positive baby is usually born before the immune antibodies can affect its cells, but the continued ability of the mother to produce the antibodies may result in their reaction with the blood cells of a subsequent Rh-positive child. The reaction is the basis of a disease known as erythroblastosis, or hemolytic disease of the newborn. The symptoms are hemolytic jaundice which may progress to death, or sometimes fetal hydrops, that is, the accumulation of fluid in the tissues and cavities of the embryo, or even maceration of the fetus, which is then stillborn.

The underlying situation for this unfortunate occurrence is, of course, an Rh-negative mother who has been immunized against the Rh factor; an Rh-positive father; and an Rh-positive child who has inherited the Rh factor from the father. The immunization of the Rh-negative mother is ordinarily the result of having previously born one or more Rh-positive children, but it may be the result of a previous transfusion with Rh-positive blood cells, in which case even the first Rh-positive child might be affected.

Levine's demonstration that the mothers of children with hemolytic disease were Rh negative led to the puzzling discovery that not all such mothers possessed antibodies in their serums demonstrable by the usual tests. This in turn led to the demonstration by Wiener, Diamond, and others that there are two types of antibodies capable of production by such mothers: bivalent, reacting to the usual saline agglutination tests; and univalent, reacting only in the presence of serum or other protein.

These facts in their turn paved the way to the important finding that not all mothers of children with hemolytic disease were producing antibodies against the original Rh factor, but that some of them exhibited antibodies against similar but different antigens. Each of these antigens appeared capable on occasion of causing, through its reaction with its own antibody, hemolytic disease in an infant, or transfusion reactions in a recipient. Each antigen occurs with its own unique frequency in the population, and each is directly inherited.

Wiener found in this way two new antigens closely related to Rh. He renamed the original factor Rh_0, calling the new ones rh′ and rh″. Levine discovered a similar antigen reciprocally related to rh′ in such a way that everyone has one or the other or both of these factors, but no one lacks both. This new reciprocal antigen he named, appropriately enough, hr.

By this time research on such antigens had spread all over the world. Fisher, in England, noting the reciprocal relationship of Levine's hr to Wiener's rh′, suggested that similar reciprocal antigens would be found to Rh_0 and rh″. This prediction has been fulfilled. Still other alternate reciprocal antigens in the Rh-Hr series have been described, until now ten members of this series are known. Wiener has presented strong evidence that these ten antigens are inherited on the basis of a single set of multiple alleles.

Acting similarly to the Rh-Hr factors as far as hemolytic reactions are concerned, but genetically quite unrelated to them, are several newly described antigens which are thus far named only for the person whose cells gave rise to the antibody production. Thus we have the Kell antigen and the Cellano antigen, reciprocally related to each other but independent of the rest; the Lewis antigen, the Lutheran antigen, and the Levay antigen.

Of the fifteen known antigens of the third category, only the original Rh_0 appears to initiate antibody production strongly enough and often enough to be of real clinical significance. This antigen is the one which stimulated the production of antibodies in nearly all the recorded instances of hemolytic disease and in almost all the severe transfusion reactions. However, inasmuch as the other antigens of this category were originally discovered by virtue of their clinical manifestations, they cannot be completely ignored from the clinical standpoint, even though they are of far less significance than Rh_0.

Some recent work indicates that occasionally immunization of a mother by one of these antigens results in manifestations of still other sorts: mental deficiency, congenital anomalies, and the like. Current research in progress in various parts of the world, as yet reported only in personal communications, seems to confirm this in some instances and to deny it in others. The final outcome must await the future.

In any event, a married woman expecting her first child should most certainly be tested for Rh_0. If she is negative and her husband positive, the obstetrician will be in a position to take such steps as may be available for depressing the formation of antibodies and for minimizing or counteracting their possible effects on the child. Effective means for bringing about these desirable results are gradually coming to hand.

The final portion of this paper deals with a frontier of

which genetics is not proud, but which has been forced upon it by a political frontal attack. Pushing back the boundaries of the unknown is a stimulating experience; defending the ground thus won against aggression involving weapons long since thought to be outlawed in scientific discussions is depressing. Yet, inasmuch as I was asked to include a statement of the status of this frontier, I shall attempt a brief assay of the present positions.

Although the years following the overthrow of the Tsarist oppression saw a rapid and remarkable development of genetics in Russia, with the widest international exchange of ideas, this freedom of growth was short lived. As early as the mid-thirties, when plans for the Seventh International Congress of Genetics, to be held in Moscow, were still being made, the Russians stated that no session or paper dealing with human genetics could be held. Already the Russian misconception of the Western geneticists' view of the interaction of heredity and environment was making itself felt. Although Vavilov, an outstanding Russian geneticist, had been elected to the presidency of the forthcoming Congress, he was attacked for espousing "foreign" science, and the Congress was "postponed" so long that it was not held in Russia. It was held in Edinburgh in 1939, but Vavilov was not permitted to attend. He was dismissed from his post as director of the Institute of Genetics and from the presidency of the Academy of Agricultural Sciences.

These things came about largely because of the growing power of T. D. Lysenko, a follower of I. V. Michurin. Michurin was a practical plant breeder who, by virtue of a sharp eye and a long practical experience with plants, was able to select, after hybridization, several valuable varieties of fruits adapted to the severe Russian climate. Michurin also did grafting experiments and formulated the theory that the grafted stock became actually a vegetative hybrid.

Cytogenetic studies of such grafts reveal their true condition: some are chimeras, some are virus-infected transfers, and so on, but none is a true genetic hybrid. Other beliefs of Michurin, who had no biological training, have also proved indefensible when scientifically examined.

Lysenko adopted all Michurin's teachings, and added to them ideas of his own. Some of these include the virtues of "vernalization," which was not actually Lysenko's own discovery. Vernalization consists of the transformation of winter cereals into spring varieties by chilling and soaking the seeds. Much of Lysenko's fame rests on this alleged discovery, yet repetition of this practice in various parts of the world has shown it to be of very low value in comparison with standard genetic hybridization. Other experiments of Lysenko have been repeated by Western geneticists, with similar negative results. Sax states categorically that, in spite of Lysenko's claims of the practical virtues of graft hybridization, not a single authentic case is known to the scientific world.

Upon becoming president of the Academy of Agricultural Sciences, Lysenko increased the vigor of his attacks on Mendelian genetics. He ridiculed the "neat chromosome theory," stating that orthodox geneticists had made no contribution to practical agriculture. This is palpably not true, as I pointed out in the early part of this paper. Much of the verbal fireworks directed at Mendelian genetics is aimed at the genetics of thirty or forty years ago. This review will have failed its purpose if it has not made it clear that many additions and modifications have been made to the genetic principles known in 1910.

Similarly the attack on modern genetics on the ground that it assumes that heredity is completely independent of the environment loses its force in the light of discussions of this matter by leading Western geneticists over the last twenty years or more (see, for example, the Messenger Lectures presented at Cornell University in 1945 by Muller, Little, and Snyder). Every modern geneticist knows that genes and their accompanying cytoplasm do not alone make an organism. There is always an environment of some sort in which the organism develops, and which may have a greater or lesser effect on the manifestations of its characteristics and its ability to reproduce in competition with other individuals.

This does not imply, however, that acquired characters are inherited. Most Mendelian geneticists would say they are not; Lysenko insists that such inheritance is possible and necessary. He holds that any form of animal or plant can be made to change quickly and in a direction desirable to man, by purposely changing its environment.

As Wright has pointed out, an energetic attack using merely selection would quickly bring desirable results in a country with relatively unimproved livestock and cultivated plants. This would be what any orthodox geneticist would expect, and would not necessarily involve the inheritance of acquired characters.

The question of the inheritance of acquired characters, and for that matter, most of the problems at issue in the controversy, cannot be settled by preconceived notions, by philosophical debate, by executive fiat, or by a popular vote of the people. They can be settled only by gathering the observational and experimental facts, analyzing them by the scientific method, and making the results of the observations, experiments, and analyses freely available for open frank discussion by scientists everywhere. The Western democracies stand in a better light in this respect than the totalitarian states, although we in the Western world cannot yet claim perfection in this matter. For example, many pages have been written in this country condemning the

Russian decision to teach in the universities only Michurian genetics and not Mendelian genetics. I wonder, however, how easy it would be for a philosopher espousing dialectical materialism to obtain a teaching position in the philosophy department of an American university, or for a proponent of Marxian economy to be placed in a department of economics.

Orthodox geneticists were discharged from their positions in Russia for studying "bourgeois genetics." Those of us who have signed loyalty oaths and have been investigated every time we agreed to take even a consulting job in Washington or Oak Ridge may well wonder what would happen here if by chance we should wish to broaden our concepts of world affairs by subscribing to *The Daily Worker*.

In common with most geneticists, I know of no proof for the inheritance of acquired characters. Yet most of the evidence against it is of a negative sort, and a thoroughly critical study of Lamarkism is needed. If it is false, we should not have to use as our chief argument against it the assertion that seeming examples can be explained on other grounds. Critical incontrovertible evidence is essential. Certainly the Weismannian concept of complete isolation between germ plasm and somatoplasm in all organisms can no longer be held valid. Certainly the fact that directed mutations have never been produced by man does not prove that they never will be, or that nature has never produced them.

All I am trying to say is that there are certain things in the Russian controversy which we may legitimately condemn and others which suggest that we move from our glass houses before we cast stones. We may condemn, I think, the usurping by a nontechnical political bureau of the privilege of interpreting scientific observations, on the basis of need or desire, and of deciding *ex cathedra* between two hypotheses. We may legitimately condemn the official pronouncement that the most important principle in any science is the Party principle. But when we are tempted to render wholesale indictments, sometimes in the absence of the requisite scientific data, and often on emotional rather than scientific grounds, we must take great care that in so doing we do not at the same time indict ourselves.

There can be no continued social, aesthetic, or scientific progress on a mystical, metaphysical basis. Progress will result only when people, the world over, realize that it is the unique and exalted privilege of mankind alone to understand the laws of nature as they apply to man and the universe, and so to utilize them in the control of themselves and their environment as to contribute to the advancement, happiness, and welfare of all mankind.

As Muller has pointed out, this is neither complete freedom nor complete mechanism, but in the only significant sense of these terms is both at once, working in mutual harmony. The scientist alone cannot accomplish the desired result. The philosopher, the humanist, and everyone else must aid in reaching the wisest solutions to the problems of using the results of science. And while administrative fiat may determine the interpretations to be placed on scientific observations and experiments in some parts of the world, and the extent to which they are publicized, it cannot affect one iota the fundamental truths of the laws of nature, nor their discussion by free men.

REFERENCES

Auerbach, C. "Chemical Inductions of Mutations." *Proceedings of the Eighth International Congress of Genetics,* Lund, Sweden, 1949, p. 129.

Beadle, G. W. "The Gene and Biochemistry." In *Currents in Biochemical Research,* ed. D. E. Green, New York, 1946, p. 1.

—— "Genes and the Chemistry of the Organism." Chapter 6

in *Science in Progress,* ed. G. A. Baitsell, 5th ser., New Haven, 1949.

—— "Genes and Biological Enigmas." Chapter 9 in *Science in Progress,* ed. G. A. Baitsell, 6th ser., New Haven, 1949.

Bittner, J. J. "Relation of Nursing to the Extra-chromosomal Theory of Breast Cancer in Mice." *Am. J. Cancer,* XXXV (1939), 90.

Catcheside, D. G. "Genetic Effects of Radiations." In *Advances in Genetics,* ed. M. Demerec, New York, 1948, Vol. II, p. 271.

Clausen, J. "Genetics of the Climatic Races of *Potentilla glandulosa.*" *Proceedings of the Eighth International Congress of Genetics,* Lund, Sweden, 1949, p. 162.

Cotterman, C. W. "The Biometrical Approach in Human Genetics." *Am. Naturalist,* LXXVI (1942), 144.

Cotterman, C. W., and L. H. Snyder. "Tests of Simple Mendelian Inheritance in Randomly Collected Data of One and Two Generations." *J. Am. Statistical Assn.,* XXXIV (1939), 511.

Dahlberg, G. Mathematical Methods for Population Genetics. New York, 1947.

—— "Genetics of Human Populations." In *Advances in Genetics,* ed. M. Demerec, New York, 1948, Vol. II, p. 67.

Darlington, C. D. "Heredity, Development and Infection." *Nature,* CLIV (1944), 164.

Demerec, M. "Chemical Mutagens." *Proceedings of the Eighth International Congress of Genetics,* Lund, Sweden, 1949, p. 201.

Dobzhansky, T. Genetics and the Origin of Species. 2d ed. New York, 1941.

—— "Observations and Experiments on Natural Selection in Drosophila." *Proceedings of the Eighth International Congress of Genetics,* Lund, Sweden, 1949, p. 210.

Evans, R. D. "Quantitative Inferences Concerning the Genetic Effects of Radiations on Human Beings." *Science,* CIX (1949), 299.

Fisher, R. A. The Genetical Theory of Natural Selection. Oxford, 1930.

Haddow, A. "Transformation of Cells and Viruses." *Nature,* CLIV (1944), 194.

Haldane, J. B. S. New Paths in Genetics. New York, 1942.

Haldane, J. B. S. "The Rate of Mutations of Human Genes." *Proceedings of the Eighth International Congress of Genetics,* Lund, Sweden, 1949, p. 267.

Heston, W. C., M. K. Deringer, and H. B. Andervont. "Gene-Milk Agent Relationship in Mammary Tumor Development." *J. Nat. Cancer Inst.,* V (1945), 289.

Hogben, L. An Introduction to Mathematical Genetics. New York, 1946.

Irwin, M. R. "Immunogenetics." In *Advances in Genetics,* ed. M. Demerec, New York, 1947, Vol. I, p. 133.

Landsteiner, K., and A. S. Wiener. "Agglutinable Factors in Human Blood Recognized by Immune Sera for Rhesus Blood." *Proceedings of the Soc. for Experimental Biology and Medicine,* XLIII (1940), 223.

Lea, D. E. Actions of Radiations on Living Cells. Cambridge, England, 1945.

Levine, P. "A Survey of the Significance of the Rh Factor." *Blood, the J. of Hematology,* Special Issue no. 2, p. 3.

Li, Ching Chun. An Introduction to Population Genetics. Peiping, China, 1948.

Lysenko, T. The Science of Biology Today. New York, 1948.

Macklin, M. T. "The Value of Medical Genetics to the Clinician." Chapter 6 in C. B. Davenport *et al., Medical Genetics and Eugenics,* Philadelphia, 1941.

Muller, H. J. "Artificial Transmutation of the Gene." *Science,* LXVI (1927), 84.

—— "Genetics in the Scheme of Things." *Proceedings of the Eighth International Congress of Genetics,* Lund, Sweden, 1949, p. 96.

Muller, H. J., C. C. Little, and L. H. Snyder. Genetics, Medicine, and Man. Ithaca, New York, 1947.

Neel, J. V. "The Clinical Detection of the Genetic Carriers of Inherited Disease." *Medicine,* XXVI (1947), 115.

Race, R. R. "The Rh Genotypes and Fisher's Theory." *Blood, the J. of Hematology,* Special Issue No. 2, p. 27.

Rife, D. C. The Dice of Destiny. Columbus, Ohio, 1948.

Sax, K. "Genetics and Agriculture." *Bull. Atomic Scientists,* V (1949), 143.

Snyder, L. H. "Medical Genetics and Public Health: the

Twenty First Herman M. Biggs Memorial Lecture." *Bull. N. Y. Acad. Med.,* XXII (1946), 566.

—— "The Principles of Gene Distribution in Human Populations." *Yale J. Biol. and Med.,* XIX (1947), 817.

—— "The Genetic Approach to Human Individuality." *Sci. Mo.,* LXVIII (1949), 165.

—— The Principles of Heredity. 4th ed. Boston, 1951.

Sonneborn, T. M. "A New Genetic Mechanism and Its Relation to Certain Types of Cancer." *Q. Bull. Indiana Univ. Med. Center,* IX (1947), 51.

—— "Beyond the Gene," *Am. Scientist,* XXXVII (1949), 33.

Wiener, A. S. Blood Groups and Transfusion. 3d ed. Springfield, Ill., 1943.

—— "Heredity of the Rh Blood Types." *Proceedings of the Eighth International Congress of Genetics,* Lund, Sweden, 1949, p. 500.

Wright, S. "Statistical Genetics and Evolution." *Bull. Am. Math. Soc.,* XLVIII (1942), 223.

—— "Dogma or Opportunism?" *Bull. Atomic Scientists,* V (1949), 141.

MACHINES THAT WORK LIKE MEN

By John H. Gibbon Jr., M.D.

THE TITLE of this paper suggests a discussion of a mechanical automaton that in some way acts and reacts like a human being. This I am not qualified to discuss. I propose, however, to describe the present status of a mechanical contrivance which will temporarily perform the functions of the heart and lungs without harm to the subject. The title, therefore, might better be phrased as "Machines That Act Like a Heart and Lungs."

One might well ask, What is the use of a machine that acts like a heart and lungs? There are two reasons for developing and perfecting such a machine. The first is to relieve the heart and lungs of some of the work they have to do for a short period of time in an emergency. Such emergency conditions are those that happen when a diseased heart with crippled valves fails to perform its work properly under some additional strain. Another emergency is when the heart is unable temporarily to continue its pumping action, because of diminished blood supply to the heart muscle. This is the dreaded "heart failure" which is so common among "high-powered" Americans. A third emergency might be when, for some reason or another, the little air cells in the lungs become full of a watery fluid that seeps out of the blood, and the patient is actually drowning in his own fluid. Other uses for such a machine might be temporary help to blue babies while they are being operated upon, or temporary help to the heart of patients who have lost a great deal of blood. These are some of the emergencies in which a machine which could do part of the work of the heart and lungs, even for a short time, would be very helpful.

The other reason for building and perfecting such a machine is in the hope that some day it might take over the entire work of the heart and lungs for a period of time long enough to permit a surgeon to open the chambers of the heart and to perform operations inside it. Under these conditions it might be possible to correct malformations which sometimes are present at birth, or to graft in new tissue to take the place of damaged valves, which often occur as a result of rheumatic fever. At present it is impossible to open the heart and perform these operations under direct vision, because the heart is full of blood and must keep the blood circulating through the body. By-passing the blood around the heart and lungs would allow the surgeon to open the heart without losing blood and to operate in the empty inside chambers, knowing that the job of the heart and lungs was being temporarily performed by a machine.

To enable the lay person to understand what such a heart-lung machine must do, I would like to describe briefly the work performed by the human heart and lungs. There are about six quarts of blood in the body. The blood is in constant movement. In the muscles, the skin, and the other tissues of the body, it passes through tiny channels so small that they cannot be seen without magnification. Here substances are exchanged between tissues and the blood. Food is taken up by the tissues and waste products given off to the blood, but the most essential exchange that takes place between the blood and the cells concerns the breathing of the cells. They must have oxygen for their life, and carbon dioxide is the waste product which they give off in their breathing.

Any stopping of this breathing process in the cells is rapidly fatal. This is particularly true of the most highly developed cells, which are in the brain. Many of these will die if the blood supply to the brain is stopped for three or four minutes. If the blood flow is stopped for five or six minutes, the brain cells concerned with seeing are damaged, and no animal or man is able to live if the blood flow to the brain is completely stopped for ten minutes.

The reverse of this breathing process takes place in the lungs. Here the waste carbon dioxide is given off to the outside air and a new supply of oxygen from the outside air is taken up by the blood. This exchange in the lungs takes place in minute blood vessels, too small to be seen by the naked eye, which, like a net, surround little pockets of air in the lungs. The lungs are thus like two huge marine or rubber sponges. They provide a gigantic surface for exposing the blood to the air. If all the little pockets of the lung were opened up and spread out flat, they would cover an area about as large as the floor of a good-sized room.

The heart is an amazing organ. It never stops working from the time we are born till we die. A partition divides the heart into two parts which have no direct communication with each other. The right side of the heart receives the dark blood that comes back from the tissues and pumps it into the sponge-like lungs. The bright red blood, which has changed color because it has picked up oxygen in the lungs, returns through the veins of the lungs to the left side of the heart. The left side then pumps this red arterial blood to all the tissues of the body, supplying them with oxygen. Each side of the heart pumps an exactly equal amount of blood, which amounts to about four quarts a minute.

Two other facts about blood should be understood. One is that about half of the blood consists of tiny microscopic cells which hold hemoglobin, the substance that allows the cells to pick up a large amount of oxygen. The other fact of importance is that whenever blood escapes from a blood vessel and is exposed to air it changes within a few minutes from a liquid into a solid jelly. This feature protects us from bleeding to death whenever we cut a finger on a tin can—one of the hazards of modern living.

Now, to do the work of the heart and lungs we must have two pumps and a mechanical lung. One pump will draw blood out of the great veins of the body before it gets to the heart and pump this blood into the mechanical lung. The second pump will return the blood from the mechanical lung to the blood vessels on the other side of the heart (these are called arteries), thus by-passing the heart and lungs and doing their work. The mechanical lung must provide a huge filming surface and yet must be reasonably compact. The passage of the blood through the mechanical heart and lungs must be done without damaging the tiny red blood cells, and the blood must be prevented from clotting while passing through the mechanical heart and lungs. When the normal heart and lungs again take over their job, the blood must recover its normal clotting ability.

Our apparatus * consists of two pumps and a large vertical cylinder which performs the job of the lungs. The apparatus is enclosed in an air-conditioned cabinet to keep the blood at body temperature. The first pump draws blood from the experimental subject and plays it against the inside surface, at the top, of the large revolving cylinder. Centrifugal force

* This was constructed for us by the International Business Machines Corporation, through the generosity of Thomas J. Watson, Chairman of the Board.

causes the blood to be spread out on the inner surface of the cylinder in a thin film. Oxygen is blown over this film, which absorbs oxygen and gives off carbon dioxide. The blood is collected in a cup at the bottom of the cylinder. From this cup the red blood is pumped back into the arteries of the subject. Thus, one pump corresponds to, and does the work of, the right side of the heart; the vertical cylinder performs the work of the lungs; and the other pump acts as the left side of the heart in pumping oxygenated blood from the lungs to the rest of the body.

Before any such machine as this can be used for human beings, it must be tried out again and again on animals, to make sure that it can do no harm and will, indeed, be of help to patients who need it. The machine that we have developed, and on which we are still working, is large enough and efficient enough now to take over the work of the heart and lungs in dogs. It is these experiments that I will now describe.

In our first experiments our aim was to pump blood continuously out of a dog's vein, pass it through our mechanical lung, and then pump it back into the arteries. We knew we were only pumping a part of the circulation through our machine, the rest was going through the dog's own heart and lungs in the ordinary way. When we were able to do this successfully in six consecutive experiments for periods up to two and a half hours, and have the six dogs live afterward in a perfectly normal healthy condition, we were satisfied that it did no harm to take over a part of the work of the heart and lungs by a mechanical apparatus.

Next we had to show that the apparatus was capable of doing *all* the work of a dog's heart and lungs: that it could keep the dog alive while no blood at all was going through its heart, and that it could recover in a perfectly healthy condition after short periods of such "artificial circulation."

Our dogs were anesthetized with general anesthesia, sterile drapes and instruments were laid out, and the doctor and his assistant "scrubbed up," just as is done in all human operations. After the dog was asleep, two small incisions were made in the thighs, over the arteries that supply blood to the legs. The incisions were just big enough to give access to the femoral arteries, so that we could tie a cannula into each artery; one cannula was for the purpose of returning the blood from our machine to the dog and the other was connected to a manometer, on which was recorded the blood pressure of the dog throughout the experiment.

Next, an opening was made in the chest, and now it was necessary to use artificial respiration, to inflate and deflate the lungs while the chest was open to the air. In order to draw blood from the great veins before it reached the heart, cannulas were inserted in such a way that their open ends projected into the superior and inferior venae cavae. These cannulas were connected with tubing to the first pump of our apparatus.

Meanwhile, the apparatus had been filled with blood from a donor dog and, when all the preparations were completed, the blood of our experimental dog was rendered temporarily incoagulable by adding to it by injection a small amount of heparin, which prevents blood from clotting when exposed to air. Then a stopcock in the circuit was opened and the apparatus began to draw blood from the cannulas in the big veins near the heart. The blood was pumped from the dog onto the inner surface of the rapidly revolving cylinder; there it was spread out in a very thin film. Oxygen was continuously blown over this film of blood as it ran down the sides of the cylinder and the blood, now bright red, was collected in the glass cup at the bottom of the cylinder. From here our second pump took the blood to the cannula in the dog's leg artery, whence it was pumped up through the large vessel (the aorta), to the heart. Here a valve prevented it from flowing into the heart; instead it flowed out of the branches of the aorta, just as it does normally, carrying its supply of oxygen to all parts of the body.

After half an hour or more, the machine was stopped; the cannulas were taken out of the veins and arteries; the chest was closed, and the skin incisions sewed together. Another drug was injected into the dog's blood, to counteract the nonclotting effect of the heparin, because now it was important to have the blood able to clot normally, so that the animal would not bleed from his wounds. Usually, the dog woke up in a few hours, and in twenty-four hours it was able to eat and drink. In a few days it appeared entirely recovered and normal. In each case, the dog was then kept in the laboratory and observed for several months. As of this writing, most of these experimental dogs have been adopted and have become pampered pets in various homes.

BIOLOGICAL ASPECTS OF ANTIBIOTICS *

By Selman A. Waksman, Ph.D.

INTRODUCTION BY THE CHAIRMAN (René J. Dubos, Rockefeller Institute of Medical Research): Among American men of science, there is none whose name is more familiar to the medical and lay public than that of Selman Waksman. Dr. Waksman was born in Kiev, Russia, on July 2, 1888, and became an American citizen half a century ago. His struggles as a student and as a laboratory worker in California and New Jersey, his discovery of the spectacular drug streptomycin have been publicized in newspapers and on the radio all over our land; indeed, all over the world. His portrait in color has appeared on the cover of *Time* magazine—truly the epitome of recognition and fame in these United States.

It would seem, therefore, as if nothing were left to tell concerning him. And yet, the most interesting has been left unsaid. What I wish to evoke are the unsung labors and trials of a life devoted to science—to pursuits for which there was no indication that they would ever yield popular rewards. For more than three decades Dr. Waksman dedicated himself to the study of the complex and mysterious

* From a Journal Series Paper, New Jersey Agricultural Experiment Station, Rutgers University, The State University of New Jersey, Department of Microbiology.

processes by which the organic substances in soil, in water, in all natural environments, undergo an eternal cycle of chemical transformation through the agency of microbial life. The knowledge that he thus acquired of all microscopic living things, of their manifold chemical activities and of their competitive behavior and inter-relationships, prepared him for the discovery in soil of microorganisms capable of destroying disease-producing germs. The end result of Dr. Waksman's theoretical investigations has been of obvious use in the control of disease. It is for this reason that the world acclaims him today. But, to some of us who were associated with him before, there is even greater romance in having known him as the tireless student of all living things that populate the microscopic world.

Streptomycin and its glamor are familiar to all of you and need no introduction. In the name of a past equally brilliant, although less well known, and speaking for hundreds of his students all over the world, I am happy to introduce my teacher of twenty-five years ago, Dr. Selman A. Waksman, microbiologist of the New Jersey Experimental Station.

THE ABILITY of certain microorganisms to inhibit the growth of other organisms and, from an even broader point of view, the ability of certain living cells to inhibit the growth of other cells have such wide and fundamental implications that we must consider their significance from every possible angle. Numerous theories have been proposed to explain these effects of growth inhibition of one cell upon another. It is now generally agreed that this is due largely, at least in the case of the microorganisms, to the production of certain chemical compounds which are active in very dilute solutions and which we designate as "antibiotics."

INTRODUCTORY NOTE

Had I been invited to present a paper on this topic ten years ago, I would, no doubt, have considered within the space allowed to me, all that was known about antibiotics and had some space to spare. Within the last decade, however, there has grown up a new field of science, with its biological, chemical, and chemotherapeutic implications. This new science not only has broadened greatly our concept of the growth and activities of microorganisms, it not only has led to the isolation of many new compounds and, one might say, to a new concept in medicinal chemistry and to creation of a new pharmaceutical industry, but it has also revolutionized medical practice and has placed in the hands of the physician powerful tools for combating numerous infectious diseases that appeared, only a few years ago, to be completely unconquerable by chemotherapy. It is hardly possible at the present time, in the scope of a single address, to do more than draw a broad outline of the subject of antibiotics, directing attention to the background that led to its development, and limiting myself largely to the biological aspects of this rapidly developing subject.

In addressing the National Academy of Sciences in Washington on April 18, 1940, I said:

> Bacteria pathogenic for man and animals find their way to the soil, either in the excreta of the hosts or in their remains. If one considers the period for which animals and plants have existed on this planet and the great numbers of disease-producing microbes that must have thus gained entrance into the soil, one can only wonder that the soil harbors so few bacteria capable of causing infectious diseases in man and in animals. One hardly thinks of the soil as a source of epidemics. What has become of all the bacteria causing typhoid, dysentery, cholera, diphtheria, pneumonia, bubonic plague, tuberculosis, leprosy, and numerous others? This question was first raised

by medical bacteriologists in the eighties of the last century. The soil was searched for bacterial agents of infectious diseases, until the conclusion was reached that these do not survive long in the soil. It was suggested that the cause of the disappearance of these disease-producing organisms in the soil is to be looked for among the soil-inhabiting microbes, antagonistic to the pathogens and bringing about their rapid destruction in the soil.

This prophecy was fully justified. Only six years later, there was held in this very city, at the New York Academy of Sciences, a three-day conference on antibiotics. In addressing this conference, I said:

> The coordinated efforts of the microbiologist, the chemist, the pharmacologist, and the clinician will finally lead to the control of these and many other diseases that are now plaguing mankind. The microbiologist will have made his contribution, by the isolation of new microbes capable of forming non-toxic substances active against various disease-producing organisms; by developing methods for the optimum growth of these organisms and for measuring their antibacterial activities; by helping to elucidate the mode of action of antibiotics upon the disease-causing agents; and, finally, by evaluating the practical potentialities of antibiotic substances as chemotherapeutic agents.

To complete this brief survey and to reemphasize the rapid development of the subject of antibiotics, I may mention that only three and a half years later, in June, 1949, another conference was held under the auspices of the same society, but now dealing with only one narrow phase of the subject, namely, the chemotherapy of tuberculosis. Here, I said:

> Chemotherapy of tuberculosis has made tremendous progress during the last decade. I might be so bold as to say that ten years ago one could hardly dare to mention this subject before a scientific or medical gathering, except in a mere whisper, for fear of being declared a visionary. On April 21 of this year, I

attended a conference arranged by the Veterans Administration in Denver where four days were devoted to a discussion of streptomycin in tuberculosis. The enthusiasm aroused was unlimited, and the general feeling was that we were rapidly approaching the time when chemotherapy of tuberculosis will become a reality.

Two other important conferences held in Washington under the auspices of the Antibiotic Study Section of the United States Public Health Service, in 1946 and in 1949, bear further evidence of the rapid growth of this field of science and of its numerous applications, both theoretical and applied.

No wonder, therefore, that antibiotics are viewed in the popular mind as "miracle drugs" and that the medical profession speaks of this period as the "antibiotic age." This is illustrated by an editorial in the American Journal of Medicine, written by Dr. Tillett, who says:

> It has been an exciting era that has seen a drop in the mortality. The veering of emphasis which has resulted from antibiotic therapy may be seen in surgical management in which patients are well saturated with antibacterial reagents before, during and after operative procedures. In viewing the antibiotic age, perhaps greater interest, even if of a more speculative nature, centers around whether or not the present-day satisfaction with the success of antibacterial therapy can be transformed into a permanent optimism for generations to come.

HISTORICAL DATA

In analyzing this rapid growth of the science of antibiotics, one is inclined to wonder whether the progress that has been made during such a brief period has come out like Venus fully matured from the head of Zeus or whether there was a long preparatory period in which many uncoordinated observations were made, which gradually formed a solid basis for its sudden outburst. A mere cursory observation of the literature (see Waksman, 1937–1949, in list of references) will convince us that the latter is the case.

Folklore abounds in illustrations of the use of microbes or of their products for repression of microbial infections or for preventing infections. I receive numerous letters drawing my attention to the use of a variety of materials, such as cheese, stable manure, compost materials, for the treatment of boils and of similar infections. "Whenever I cut myself as a child," writes a lady of Polish extraction, "my mother used to hurry to the attic and bring down some cobwebs and cover up the wound." "Whenever I was wounded," writes a gentleman from the Pennsylvania Dutch country, "my mother would take some well-ripened cheese and cover up the wound." A farmer from the Cameron country wrote that "Witch doctors treat their patients by feeding them earth. Why not study that particular earth?"

These popular concepts found a practical application on a much larger scale under very special circumstances. This can be illustrated by the following observations:

1. Certain practices of surgery are based upon the creation of conditions favorable to the development of antagonistic microorganisms; during the Spanish Civil War, the method of cast surgery or plaster treatment of wounds was introduced; the saprophytic bacterial flora prevented infection of the wounds; the only objectionable part of this method of treatment was the putrefactive smells that such wounds produced.

2. Mixed infections were often milder than pure infections; this fact was often used for the control of serious diseases as by applying less pathogenic organisms or saprophytic organisms in the treatment of infections like anthrax or tuberculosis.

3. When polluted water contains cells of the *pyocyaneus* organism, the *typhoid* bacillus will never have a chance to develop or at least will not show its presence in the water, as determined by the presumptive tests.

4. Certain soils were frequently spoken of as immune to specific pathogens, such as "cholera-immune."

The bacteriologist and the chemist also made some very striking observations bearing upon the antagonistic effects of microorganisms. As long ago as 1877, Pasteur noticed that the growth of certain air-borne organisms inhibited growth of the anthrax bacillus. He suggested that this fact might be of importance in therapeutics. About the same time, Tyndall carried out experiments on the effect of certain molds upon the growth of bacteria. He emphasized the absence of uniformity manifested in the struggle for existence between the bacteria and the penicillia. In some tubes the former were triumphant; in other tubes of the same infusion the latter were triumphant.

Fleming commented on these observations as follows:

> It is certain that every bacteriologist has not once but many times had culture plates contaminated with moulds. It is also probable that some bacteriologists have noticed similar changes to those noted above, but that, in the absence of any special interest in naturally occurring antibacterial substances, the cultures have simply been discarded. It was, however, fortunate that . . . I was always on the lookout for new bacterial inhibitors, and when I noticed on a culture plate that the staphylococcal colonies in the neighborhood of a mould had faded away I was sufficiently interested in the antibacterial substance produced by the mould to pursue the subject.

With an increase in our knowledge of the influence of nutrition and environment upon the growth and activities of pathogenic organisms within and without the host, a better appreciation was developed of the antagonistic effects of one organism upon another. Numerous references are found in the literature to the formation of specific compounds, which were designated as bacterolysins, bactericidal agents, toxic factors, lethal principles, and others. All were products of microbial life, and all had the capacity of destroying, in one way or another, microbes with which they came in contact. The mechanism of such action was not always sufficiently understood. It was often confused with the action of cells of the same microbe upon one another or upon closely related forms, or with enzyme or lytic mechanisms, or with nutritional problems.

The various theories suggested at one time or another to explain the mechanism of growth inhibition of one organism by another can be summarized as follows:

Exhaustion of nutrients
Physicochemical changes in medium
Pigment action
Action at a distance
Space antagonism
Enzyme action, either directly by the antagonist or as a result of cell autolysis, under the influence of the antagonist
Production and liberation of antibiotic substances

Although it was becoming gradually recognized that the last theory, the production of antibiotics by one organism that has a growth-inhibiting or destructive effect upon another, forms the basis for all, or at least most, of these activities, the significance of these substances in nature and especially their use as chemotherapeutic agents was hardly recognized.

It is true that a great variety of microbial products were previously utilized, or at least efforts had been made to utilize them, in the treatment of various infections. Beginning with Cantani in 1893 and ending with Rappin in 1912 and Vaudremer in 1913, either living cells of microorganisms or macerations of living or dead cells were utilized in the treatment of tuberculosis. The results obtained were either inconclusive or unreproducible, and at best were only insufficiently understood. The same may be said of the one antibiotic that was known for more than half a century and used for practical control of disease more than any of the others, namely, pyocyanase. For a number of reasons, such as instability of preparation, lack of knowledge of its mode of action upon bacteria, the ability of *B. pyocyaneus* to produce several different antibiotics, and an insufficient appreciation of the fact that one was dealing here not with an isolated phenomenon but with a widely distributed system of biological activities, pyocyanase never came into its own. It must, therefore, be relegated to the limbo of forgotten or misplaced discoveries, like such other antibiotics as mycophenolic acid, the first antibiotic ever isolated from fungus cultures, the lysozyme-like materials produced by actinomycetes, and the various products of spore-forming bacteria, notably those of *B. subtilis* and of *B. mycoides*.

Many other observations pointed to the existence of various mechanisms produced by certain microorganisms and responsible for the destruction of other organisms. Attention has already been called to the fact that the soil has long been known as the major burial ground for many pathogenic organisms, but still, with certain rare exceptions, it never becomes a source of infections and epidemics. Enrichment of soil with pathogenic organisms has actually been used for the purpose of isolating bactericidal substances in order to combat disease-producing bacteria. This procedure led to the isolation of a group of antibiotics now known as the tyrothricin complex.

Experience in plant pathology also offers many illustrations of the production by some organism of mechanisms destructive to others. Although in many cases such phenomena were ascribed to the rather vague concept of "staling," in others attempts have been made to isolate the agents concerned and even to utilize them for disease control. This is true, for example, of the gliotoxin isolated by Weindling from cultures of various fungi, of the factor produced by *Bacillus simplex,* studied by Haensler and his students and later described as simplexin, and of the many studies of Russian investigators on the "bacterization" of seeds to prevent their infection by pathogenic fungi.

Another illustration of antagonistic effects of microorganisms, although somewhat indirect, is found in the investigations on the replacement, in the intestinal canal, of one bacterial flora by another, either by special method of nutrition or by actual consumption of bacterial cells. This concept, originated under such auspices as Metchnikov, contributed little to our knowledge of antibiotics, but it tended to clarify greatly the idea of existing bacterial populations. *Escherichia coli* has been used for replacing pathogenic bacteria in the gut. In the treatment of diphtheria organisms, recourse was had to use of certain bacteria, such as lactic acid organisms or *Staphylococcus aureus;* the resulting effects were not always favorable to the host. Use of various forms of yeasts, by different methods of administration, also had a certain popularity at one time, with uncertain results. Cultures of lactobacilli were used for both internal and external administration, as in the treatment of vaginal trichomoniasis. Cultures of *Lactobacillus acidophilus* are said to be beneficial in the treatment of various forms of diarrhea and dysentery.

Numerous efforts to replace in the soil a given population by another artificially introduced led to rather discouraging results, unless accompanied simultaneously by a change in soil management, as by liming of soil, adding stable manures, or growing leguminous or other host plants.

In spite of this extensive background of knowledge of antagonistic effects of microorganisms and in spite of a growing recognition that certain organisms are capable of affecting the growth of others and thus modifying if not completely suppressing the disease caused by them, no clear concept of the significance and of the tremendous potentialities of this field was obtained until about a decade ago. There were many facts and uncoordinated observations. A synthesis of the whole field was required, and marvelous fruit would come forth as from the horn of the goddess. This occurred in 1939. Announcement of the isolation of gramicidin and tyrocidine was the stimulus which flooded with bright light the whole previously unillumined field, and which was to set in motion the whole marvelous plan of study and application of antibiotics. This was to be followed by numerous new discoveries, and many of the previous observations, which remained unclear and unappreciated, were also becoming clarified.

NATURE AND FORMATION OF ANTIBIOTICS

The word "antibiotic" has had an old and varied usage. This ranged from the dictionary concept of "anything that inhibits life" to the recent and somewhat loose idea of "antibiotic therapy," which includes the use of antibiotics in therapy, on the one extreme, to any form of therapy in which chemical agents are employed, on the other. The tendency has also been to broaden the term to include all substances of biological origin which possess antimicrobial properties. To attach proper significance to the term, a redefinition at this time is justified:

An antibiotic is a product of microbial life which has the capacity of inhibiting and even of destroying, in dilute solutions, various microorganisms.

Quinine is thus not an antibiotic, since it is produced by plants; neither is lysozyme, since it is an animal product. Alcohol is not an antibiotic, since it acts in concentrated solutions, nor are the sulfonamides, since they are synthetic products. Penicillin, streptomycin, and tyrothricin are typical antibiotics, since they are produced by fungi, actinomycetes, and bacteria, respectively, and have the capacity of inhibiting growth of various bacteria in very dilute solutions. Dihydrostreptomycin is an antibiotic derivative, since it is produced from an antibiotic and acts in a manner similar to the substance from which it was derived. Chloromycetin is an antibiotic, despite its present synthetic production, because it is formed by a microorganism and was first so obtained.

The ability to produce antibiotics is widely distributed among microorganisms. However, it is not a generic or even a specific characteristic, but is limited to certain strains within a given species. The variation in the production of antibiotics is both quantitative and qualitative. Strains of *Penicillium notatum* and of *P. chrysogenum* vary in their capacity to form penicillin between less than 1 unit and more than 1,000 units per 1 ml. of culture medium. The composition of medium and the conditions of cultivation greatly influence the amount and even the nature of the penicillin produced. Various strains of *S. griseus* differ greatly in their ability to form streptomycin: some give rise also to other antibiotics, such as actidione and streptocin; some form no streptomycin, but only other antibiotics; whereas some form no antibiotics at all. The problem is thus not only to find a given organism which forms a certain antibiotic, but also to find one that produces the particular antibiotic in sufficient concentrations to justify its practical manufacture.

Among the important properties of antibiotics is their capacity to act selectively upon certain bacteria. Some antibiotics act largely upon gram-positive bacteria, some act upon gram-negative bacteria, others act upon bacteria within each of these groups, and still others act upon rickettsiae and the larger viruses; some act upon fungi, upon trichomonads, or upon trypanosomes. Each antibiotic is thus characterized by a specific antibiotic spectrum, namely, its selective quantitative and qualitative effect upon different microorganisms.

Upon contact with a certain antibiotic, various bacteria may develop resistance to it. This is because a given bacterial culture is made up of many cells which vary greatly in their sensitivity to the antibiotic. The more sensitive cells are killed off, and the more resistant ones gradually give rise to a new population of bacteria which are more resistant than the original culture. This process is accompanied by a change in a certain biochemical mechanism of the bacterial culture, which is concerned with the synthesis of the cell material by the bacteria. In some cases, strains of bacteria are obtained which become dependent upon the presence of the antibiotic for their growth.

Although nearly 200 antibiotics are now recognized, only very few have found practical application as chemotherapeutic agents. Among the bacterial products may be listed tyrothricin, bacitracin, polymyxin, and nisin. Among the fungus products, only penicillin is used. Among the products of actinomycetes, streptomycin, aureomycin, chloromycetin, and possibly neomycin may be listed.

Numerous laboratories throughout the world are now engaged in a search for new antibiotics. Many soils and other natural substrates are used for this purpose. Before a new antibiotic can qualify as a chemotherapeutic agent, it must fulfill certain definite requirements, which can be briefly summarized as follows:

1. It must be selective in action against various organisms, and should not be a generalized protoplasmic poison.

2. It must have desirable antibacterial properties, that is, it must affect bacteria or other microorganisms that are not subject to the action of another antibiotic, or it must be more potent or more effective than another which is to be replaced.

3. It must exert not only a bacteriostatic but also a bactericidal effect upon microorganisms.

4. It should not be reduced in its potency by the body fluids or be destroyed by tissue enzymes.

5. It should not be toxic in concentrations used for combating infections.

6. It should not damage leucocytes in concentrations required to affect the infectious bacteria or be injurious to the kidneys and to other body tissues.

7. It should possess certain desirably physical and chemical properties, such as solubility in water and a certain degree of stability.

8. It should be excreted readily from the animal system and not accumulate there and produce undesirable aftereffects.

9. It should be active in the treatment of specific infections, preferably those that are not susceptible to the action of any known drug.

10. A new antibiotic may have a synergistic effect with another one, even if it does not by itself form an ideal chemotherapeutic agent.

New antibiotics are being discovered at a very rapid rate. The names used to designate them are usually derived from the generic or the specific names of the organisms producing them, as penicillin and notatin, streptomycin and grisein, bacillin and subtilin; from the organisms acted upon, as gramicidin, borellidin, antimycin; from some chemical structure in the molecules of the antibiotics, such as actidione, chloromycetin, sulfactin, mannosidostreptomycin; from their modes of action, as mycolysin, subtilysin; from the modes of their formation, as endosubtilysin; from their pigmentation, as pyocyanin, xanthomycin; or from a combination of two properties, such as origin and activity, as flavicidin, gliotoxin. The bewildering array of designations frequently has led to confusion, especially when one remembers the fact that certain organisms produce more than one antibiotic and that the same antibiotic may be produced by several organisms. The antibiotic produced by *Aspergillus clavatus* has been given five names, depending on the organism producing it; the oxidative enzyme produced by *P. notatum*, and considered at one time to be an antibiotic, has received a number of designations.

The formation of several antibiotics by one organism may lead to confusing terminology as long as the chemical entities have not been separated from one another. As long as one is still dealing with crude preparations—and most antibiotics have been studied or at least designated when still in a crude state—one is never certain of their identifying characteristics, whether they are concerned with the chemical properties, antimicrobial activities, or toxic manifestations in the animal body. No wonder, therefore, that many chemists have suggested that no new antibiotic be given a definite name until its chemical nature has been established, and that the name be so selected as to give reference to it. In view of the fact, however, that the early stages of antibiotic research are carried out by microbiologists and that often a considerable time may elapse between the recognition of an antibiotic and the elucidation of its chemical structure—in the case of penicillin it was a spread of nearly fifteen years—this recommendation could hardly be accepted by the microbiologists.

It has now been well established that antibiotics represent a great number of chemical compounds which differ in their solubility, their chemical composition and structure, their toxicity, and their ability to inhibit the growth of different microorganisms *in vitro* and *in vivo*. Some organisms, notably various filamentous fungi, produce relatively simple antibiotics, made up of carbon, hydrogen, and oxygen, having a relatively broad antimicrobial spectrum and acting more like generalized protoplasmic poisons. Next come the organisms that produce the somewhat more complex antibiotics which contain the elements nitrogen, or nitrogen and sulfur. These vary in composition and in their antimicrobial spectra. Here belong many fungi and actinomycetes, which produce some of the most valuable chemotherapeutic agents known at present. Then come the organisms which form complex polypeptides, namely, the spore-forming bacteria. Finally, certain organisms, notably *E. coli,* give rise to a series of antibiotics which differ from one another in their selective activity upon different bacteria; whether the active preparation comprises several agents or a single compound with a variety of active groups is still to be determined.

MODE OF ACTION OF ANTIBIOTICS

Among the most fascinating problems that have arisen in connection with the study of antibiotics is their mode of action upon bacteria and the development of resistance among bacteria to antibiotics. One may also include here the formation of strains of bacteria, exposed to certain antibiotics like streptomycin, which become dependent upon these antibiotics for their growth. Although none of these problems has yet been solved satisfactorily, sufficient experimental evidence has been submitted to justify certain broad generalizations. It has now been definitely established that the sensitivity of a bacterial cell to a certain antibiotic is closely related to cell growth and multiplication, both of which depend on cell synthesis and metabolism. The fact that most of the known enzyme mechanisms, such as the diastatic, proteolytic, lipolytic, are not affected by the majority of antibiotics points to their activity on certain intermediary metabolic reactions which leads to cell synthesis rather than to energy liberation. Different antibiotics affect different mechanisms, the nature of the cell and the age of the cell being very important in this connection.

Different antibiotics vary greatly in the degree of development of bacterial resistance. S. *aureus* was found to develop marked resistance to grisein and to streptomycin, intermediate resistance to penicillin and pyocyanin, less resistance to aureomycin and neomycin, and apparently none to aspergillic acid. When the organism was made resistant to penicillin, its biochemical reactions were lost, the cells becoming pleomorphic and gram-negative. When it was made resistant to streptomycin, its characteristic biochemical reactions were also suppressed, but there was no noticeable change in its morphology.

Various explanations have been suggested for the development of resistance. These may be summarized as follows: (a) sensitive cells in a given bacterial population are killed, thereby enabling the more resistant cells to grow selectively; (b) more resistant mutants are formed in a sensitive population of bacteria; (c) acquisition of new enzyme systems or new metabolic activities permit the organism to survive in spite of the presence of the particular growth-inhibiting agent. Demerec reported that resistance of *S. aureus* to penicillin originates through a mutation mechanism and that the antibiotic acts as a selective agent to eliminate the nonresistant members of the bacterial population. The degree of resistance can be increased by selection, this increase being more rapid with each selection step.

In the development of resistance by bacteria to streptomycin, two types of variants are produced. One appears in small numbers in all concentrations of the antibiotic. It gives rise to cultures which grow both in streptomycin-free and in streptomycin-containing media, its virulence for animals being similar to that of the original strain. The second appears in greatest numbers in concentrations of streptomycin between 100 and 400 Mg./ml. This type becomes dependent upon the presence of streptomycin in the medium. It does not grow in media containing less than 5 Mg./ml. of the antibiotic and it is nonvirulent unless the animal receives streptomycin. Various cultures of bacteria produce both "resistant" and "dependent" variants. The critical concentrations of streptomycin above which the sensitive strains do not grow are about the same as those below which the dependent variants do not grow. This tends to confirm the concept that antibiotics act as metabolite antagonists, streptomycin interfering with some essential metabolite or nutritive process of the sensitive strains and serving as a growth factor for the dependent strain. This relation can be reversible for the dependent strains, but it is permanent in the case of the resistant strains.

ANTIBIOTICS AND LIFE

Finally, we come to the question of the significance of antibiotics in nature. The first impulse would naturally be to ascribe to them a sort of willful or protective mechanism against other microorganisms. A detailed analysis of some of the relationships involved tend to emphasize the fact, however, that this is not actually the case. It is important to remember that most of the antibiotic-producing organisms have been isolated from the soil. It is, therefore, sufficient to examine the interrelationships among soil microorganisms to determine whether such preconceived ideas are justified. Formation of penicillin and streptomycin may serve as illustrations.

Penicillin is produced by a fungus when growing in pure culture, in a highly selective medium which is rich in glucose, corn steep liquor, and other materials. The soil hardly presents such a nutritive medium for penicillin production, and is far from being a pure culture. Under the best conditions, only traces of penicillin could be formed in the soil. Since penicillin is readily destroyed by various bacteria and since these are found abundantly in the soil, this antibiotic, even if traces were formed in the soil, would probably be very rapidly destroyed there by the bacteria. Finally, and most important of all, penicillin is not effective against fungi and most of the gram-negative bacteria, both of which comprise a large portion of the soil population and against which the penicillin-producing *Penicillium notatum* would have to compete for nutrients. Hence, of what importance can penicillin be to the organism producing it in its struggle for existence?

Streptomycin presents a somewhat different group of problems. This is a stable compound and is not destroyed by other organisms. For its production, however, a protein-rich medium is required. Even if only a few cells of bacteria should find their way into a big tank where the *Streptomyces griseus* is growing, such bacteria would multiply so rapidly as to present streptomycin formation. In the soil where only very few cells of *S. griseus* are present, as compared to the vast microbiological population, and still fewer of those cells are able to produce streptomycin, what would one expect, therefore, to occur, especially when the soil contains only a limited number of nutrients required for streptomycin production? Streptomycin is not effective against fungi. Finally, all the bacteria and actinomycetes that are sensitive to it can readily adjust themselves to it. Hence, even if streptomycin were produced in the soil, its microbiological population would have long ago adapted itself to the antibiotic which would no longer have any effect upon the microbes. Of what potential importance can this agent be to the organism producing it in its competition for nutrients?

Similar reasoning can apply to most of the other antibiotics. If an antibiotic is of help to the organism producing it, we would expect that the soil would be largely inhabited by antibiotic-producing organisms. This is not the case. The ability to produce antibiotics must, therefore, be looked upon as one of those potential biological properties which the investigator discovers; he takes advantage of such properties by proper selection of strains, by development of suitable media, and by proper environmental conditions, to obtain a product which he can use to man's advantage in his own struggle for existence. The history of domestication of plants and animals offers numerous illustrations to that effect. This new branch of science, that of antibiotics, and the numerous problems and applications that have resulted, not the least important of which are the chemotherapeutic potentialities for combating human and animal infections, offer another illustration of domestication of wild forms of life for the benefit of man.

REFERENCES

Fleming, A. Penicillin and Its Practical Application. Philadelphia, 1946.

Herrell, W. E. Penicillin and Other Antibiotic agents. Philadelphia, 1945.

Irving, G. W., and H. T. Herrick. Antibiotics. Brooklyn, 1949.

Kolmer, J. A. Penicillin Therapy. New York, 1945.

Waksman, S. A. Microbial Antagonisms and Antibiotic Substances. 2d ed. New York, 1947.

—— "Antibiotics and Tuberculosis." *J. Am. Med. Assn.*, 135 (1947), 478.

—— "Antibiotics and Life." *Proceedings of the Fourth Int. Congress for Microbiology*, Copenhagen, 1947.

—— "Antibiotics." *Biol. Rev.*, 23 (1948), 452.

—— "Origin and Nature of Antibiotics." *Am. J. Med.*, 7 (1949), 85.

—— Streptomycin. Baltimore, 1949.

CONCEPTS AND METHODS OF MEDICAL RESEARCH

By Thomas M. Rivers, M.D.

SO MUCH has been said and written about the controversial subjects to be discussed tonight that I undertake the task with apprehension and humility. This is particularly true, since I cannot say anything about them that has not already been said better by many great scientists and brilliant philosophers. In addition to being controversial, the subjects are extremely important, having to do with the future well-being of man. If, then, I am fortunate enough to stimulate interest in medical research to the extent that a greater effort will be made to understand better what is going on now and what must take place in the future in this field, something will have been accomplished.

Is medical research scientific research? Before this question can be answered, one must decide whether or not medicine is a science. The Harvey Society, affiliated with The New York Academy of Medicine, was founded in 1905 with the avowed object of "The diffusion of scientific knowledge in selected chapters in anatomy, physiology, pathology, bacteriology, pharmacology, and physiological and pathological chemistry." Rufus Cole, in his Harvey Lecture in 1930, pointed out: "That medicine itself is omitted from this catalogue of sciences suggests that medicine is something different, that as an independent branch of human knowledge it does not exist, or, if so, that its content and the methods for its pursuit are not of a character to justify its inclusion in this family of sciences." Of course, Cole believes medicine to be an independent science, and in 1930 in rewriting the constitution of the Harvey Society he would have stated its object to be "the diffusion of scientific knowledge in medicine and related sciences."

Cole went on to say:

As has been pointed out, "the various branches of science are not limited by the training and antecedent interests of the persons who cultivate them, but are defined by their subject-matter." Medicine has for its subject-matter disease in its various aspects, and disease involves modification of function, but it also involves modification of structure, whether this be conceived of only in its more superficial aspects, morphology, or its more intricate nature, chemical or physical. . . . The student of disease is interested not only in describing and understanding these disturbances, but in determining the factors, intrinsic or extrinsic, on which they depend. And, just as in other sciences, even physics, its disciples are interested in obtaining accurate knowledge in order that predictions may be made, and even that the natural course of events may be modified.[1]

As late as 1945, Clark-Kennedy stated that "Medicine is not a single science, but depends on the integration of a number of sciences for the specific purpose of understanding the nature of disease as a natural phenomenon, and the application of these and other sciences to the practical problems of the prevention and treatment of ill-health." [2]

Allan Gregg in The Terry Lectures, 1941, indicated clearly his idea of medicine and its scope by the following statement concerning medical research:

1 "Progress of Medicine during the Past Twenty-five Years as Exemplified by the Harvey Society Lectures," in the *Harvey Lectures,* Baltimore, 1930, pp. 182–204.

2 A. E. Clark-Kennedy, *The Art of Medicine in Relation to the Progress of Thought,* New York, 1930, p. 6.

The uniformity of nature and the unity of science forbid us to circumscribe the content of medical research. By so much as man has a body, the methods and the knowledge of physics and chemistry are of primary importance to medical research. By so much as that body is alive, medical research finds all the fields of biology at least germane to its interests, and suggestive by analogies and comparisons. The subtleties of man's thoughts and emotions and the far reaches of his spirit . . . extend the bearing of medical research in other directions or dimensions. Nor is medical research limited at all to the study of disease. The very unity of science justifies, where, indeed, it does not enjoin, the use of any science to extend and to refine our knowledge of the substance, the behavior, in short the *nature* of man.[3]

Gregg's definition or description of medical research is elegant but, perhaps, too inclusive. The terms *clinical investigation* and *medical research* are sometimes used as though they have an identical meaning. This is not true; clinical investigation represents only a part of medical research. Medicine is a part of biology, but obviously not all of it, for many biologists have no interest whatsoever in disease. Medical investigators are of necessity interested in physiology, particularly that of human beings, but many physiologists are interested in disease only when they become personally involved in pestilences or experience ill-health. Many discoveries in physics and chemistry are of inestimable value to medicine and medical research, but that does not necessitate the inclusion of these disciplines in the science of medicine. Moreover, medical research is not the sole prerogative of physicians, witness the investigations of Pasteur, a chemist. Nor are the investigative activities of physicians limited to medicine. "Copernicus, a physician, revolutionized our ideas of the universe, but not through his profession." [4] Obviously there are different concepts of

[3] Alan Gregg, *The Furtherance of Medical Research,* New Haven, 1941, p. 2.

[4] Clark-Kennedy, p. 7.

what constitutes medicine and medical research. Resolution of these differences is not easy, and some may say that it is impossible at the present time. Nevertheless, it is essential that I try.

Even though Clark-Kennedy says that medicine is not a single science, he endows it with antiquity. According to him, Greek physicians of the Hippocratic school "broke away from preconceived ideas, and started to observe disease as an objective phenomenon of nature, keeping records of cases which are remarkable for accuracy and detail." [5] Indeed, he went so far as to say that "their great achievement was to lay the foundation of the observational method in the study of natural phenomena, and by so doing to make a contribution to science in general, and in consequence to the progress of human thought, which it would be difficult to overestimate." According to Gregg, "Medicine was the mother of the sciences in somewhat the same sense that necessity is the mother of invention." [6] Since necessity is not invention, some doubt remains as to what Gregg thinks medicine was when she gave birth to the sciences. In any event, Welch, while giving an historical sketch in 1908 of the reciprocal relations between medicine and other sciences, presented evidence to "show with what propriety medicine has been called the mother of the sciences." [7]

For the present discussion, it is not necessary to know how long medicine has been a science, nor is it essential to determine whether or not medicine was a science once upon a time, after which she fell from grace, returning only relatively recently to the elite fold. Medicine is the science that deals in the broadest sense with the understanding, prevention, and cure of disease, or, to express the same idea posi-

[5] *Ibid.* [6] Gregg, p. 38.

[7] W. H. Welch, "The Interdependence of Medicine and Other Sciences of Nature," *Science*, n.s., XXVII (1909), 49–64.

tively, medicine is the science actively involved in the understanding, maintenance, and restoration of health. Since I believe that medicine is a science, it follows that I also believe that medical research is scientific inquiry.

Since physicians, biologists, bacteriologists, immunologists, chemists, physiologists, physicists, and others have made notable contributions to the science of medicine, how does one decide whether or not the past or present activities of these different kinds of scientists constitute medical research? Frequently, it is difficult, if not impossible, to arrive at correct decisions concerning the matter. This is particularly true of the activities of many scientists no longer available for questioning. Perhaps the state of mind or attitude of the worker determines whether or not his scientific inquiry is medical, chemical, biological, bacteriological, or physiological research. If in planning his work, asking a question of nature or making an hypothesis he has the idea that the investigation to be undertaken may yield contributions, however remote, to medicine, then his activities constitute medical research.

Before scientific research and its methods are discussed, something must be said about science. By many professional and nonprofessional people, science has been divided into two kinds, pure and applied. Pure science is supposed to deal with matters of no immediate practical value, while usefulness is the keynote of applied science. However, one frequently has great difficulty in deciding whether or not one is dealing with the pure or the applied type. Cantril and associates have recently made pertinent comments concerning this matter. According to them:

> . . . It would appear that in the last analysis any scientific pursuit—no matter how abstruse it seems—is carried on because it is somehow of concern to man. Science is the human effort to understand more about nature and human nature in verifia-

ble, determined terms. The word *determined* is used here in the scientific sense as meaning high in prognostic reliability. From this it is clear that real progress in any science involves an awareness of our assumptive worlds, a consciousness of their inadequacy, and a constant, self-conscious attempt to change them so that the intellectual abstractions they contain will achieve interesting breadth and usefulness. Real progress in science means much more than merely adding to existing knowledge.[8]

In this definition of science and its interpretation, one finds the words *knowledge, understanding,* and *usefulness.* Moreover, Pasteur did not divide science into two kinds, pure and applied. He spoke of science and the application of science. This stand at least avoids what might well be a footless argument. If one agrees with Pasteur, then one would speak of medical science and its application. Thus, the activities of a practicing physician are devoted to the applications of medical science.

If one insists that there are two kinds of science, pure and applied, then there are two kinds of scientific research, pure and applied. The term *pure,* as stated before, indicates that what is being sought will, if found, add to knowledge and understanding, while *applied* means that something useful is being sought. Perhaps here, too, the attitude of the worker determines whether or not a particular piece of research is pure or applied. Of two persons working independently on the same problem, one may be conducting pure research, the other applied. In this case, the former is seeking new knowledge and more understanding without reference to usefulness, while the latter is attempting to discover something useful, caring little about the value of what he discovers in terms of new knowledge or better understanding.

[8] H. Cantril, A. Ames, Jr., A. H. Hastorf, and W. H. Ittelson, "Psychology and Scientific Research, I: The Nature of Scientific Inquiry," *Science,* CX (1949), 461–64.

Finally, both workers discover the same thing, which may or may not be useful. Immediately, many will ask: "What difference does the attitude of the worker make, so long as something is discovered?" In a certain number of instances, probably none. However, scientific research conducted by men only or primarily interested in useful results is likely to be a self-sterilizing process. For continued scientific advance, there must be sufficient investigators who place the proper value on new knowledge and increased understanding, because they themselves make advances and, through something that may be likened to catalysis, initiate and speed up work of others.

Now we come to the word *research*. One hears it so much and in connection with so many different kinds of activity that one may easily become confused and never learn its true meaning or may forget it. Indeed, on many occasions it is incorrectly used to designate certain activities in order that additional kudos will accrue to the worker, or that an undertaking may be surrounded with an aura of importance. Research is synonomous with search, investigation, or inquiry. Perhaps it is most often used to indicate a studious inquiry, or a diligent, protracted investigation. Moreover, it is not limited to scientific activities, for there are literary, antiquarian, and other kinds of research. Nor is the word *research* necessarily used to designate a re-examination, re-investigation, or a repeated search. In all kinds of research, repeated effort is often necessary to solve a problem, but, if one uses the word *research* to emphasize the repetitive nature of a search, a hyphen should be placed between the *re* and *search*. In the remarks that follow, the word *research* will be used to indicate scientific inquiry in general or such a process employed in the realm of a particular science, for example, medicine.

Scientific research is not something that comes in neat

packages, all of which have the same size, weight, and appearance. It is a process with many parts, for example, investigators, accumulated knowledge, conceptual thinking, creative imagination, hypotheses, questions, problems, insight, hunches, accidents, observation, experimentation, instruments, techniques, patience, enthusiasm, reasoning, and judgment. All of these do not necessarily play a role in every piece of research. However, some are essential and will be discussed more fully than others.

The reason for scientific research is the fact that there are problems to be solved, or questions to be answered. This, however, is not the beginning of the process, for according to Cantril and associates: "The abstractions man is able to form have on him what Dewey and Bentley characterize as a tremendous 'liberative effect,' making possible the voluntary, controlled conceptual thinking necessary for scientific inquiry and for the use of scientific method." Scientific method, however, is not scientific inquiry. Cantril and associates have made cogent remarks on this subject, and to reinforce their statements have quoted Whitehead and Einstein and Infeld. Their remarks and quotations follow:

> What we know as the scientific method is a means for pursuing scientific inquiry. If we do not bear this in mind, real progress in scientific research is apt to be thwarted. For the implicit equating of scientific inquiry and scientific method to a technique of investigation leaves out an all-important consideration: the problem of formulating a problem for scientific investigation. For the formulation of the problem for investigation must contain within itself the possibility of going beyond what is now scientifically established if it is to satisfy the definition of scentific research. . . .
>
> Whitehead [9] has pointed out that "no systematic thought has made progress apart from some adequately general working

[9] A. N. Whitehead, *Adventures of Ideas,* New York, 1933, p. 286.

hypothesis, adapted to its special topic. Such an hypothesis directs observation, and decides upon the mutual relevance of various types of evidence. In short it prescribes method."

Einstein and Infeld [10] have written that "the formulation of a problem is often more essential than its solution, which may be merely a matter of mathematical or experimental skill. To raise new questions, new possibilities, to regard old problems from a new angle, requires creative imagination and makes a real advance in science." [11]

Thus, a working hypothesis or formulation of a problem is essential to scientific research, and furthermore, the kind of hypothesis or the sort of question put to nature influences the outcome of the inquiry. Theobald Smith often remarked that a good investigator is one who asks of nature the right questions, and, according to Goldenweiser, "a scientist who is no longer capable of framing a hypothesis—or never was—is not a scientist but a methodological fossil." [12] All of this is granted, but what characterizes the scientist who can make a good hypothesis? The answer is creative imagination.

Much has been said and written about creative imagination in relation to art, literature, invention, and science. Therefore, it is obvious that the possession of this kind of imagination is not limited to scientists. In witness of its importance in science, however, is a statement by Pasteur in the recently published book on the life and work of this great man by René Dubos: "Preconceived ideas are like searchlights which illumine the path of the experimenter and serve him as a guide to interrogate nature. They be-

[10] A. Einstein and L. Infeld, The Evolution of Physics, New York, 1938, p. 95.

[11] Cantril, *et al.*, "Psychology and Scientific Research, II: Scientific Inquiry and Scientific Method," *Science,* CX (1949), 491–97.

[12] A. Goldenweiser, quoted in A. L. Porterfield, *Creative Factors in Scientific Research,* Durham, N.C., 1941, p. 112.

come a danger only if he transforms them into fixed ideas. . . . Imagination is needed to give wings to thought at the beginning of experimental investigations in any given subject."[13]

Through creative imagination a scientist constructs a working hypothesis. Then what happens? He tests the hypothesis by scientific method, which consists of observation or experimentation, or both. There are some who prefer to think of the method as observation by sampling and observation by experiment. I shall speak of it in terms of *observation* or *experimentation.*

In the infancy of most sciences, the observational method is employed exclusively, as indicated earlier in the talk by Clark-Kennedy's statement about medicine. It is usually more than just plain description of what is seen in nature, for even here a "quantitative approach" may be used, for one can weigh, measure, or count many naturally occurring objects and then subject the findings to formal mathematical treatment. The observational method, in spite of all its refinements, is held in low repute by many, for Lord Moulton remarked, "When we are reduced to observation science crawls." One should not forget, however, that a child usually crawls before it walks or runs. Observation still has a place in scientific inquiry, particularly in astronomical investigations and biological research. However, observation and recording of data without a working hypothesis are not part of scientific method. The idea that problems automatically solve themselves when sufficient observations or facts are brought together is not sound. Yet, at times, one hears that the activities of Charles Darwin support such an idea. This is not true according to Darwin's own statement

[13] René J. Dubos, *Louis Pasteur, Free Lance of Science,* Boston, 1950, p. 376.

to the effect that "collection of facts without some basis of theory for guidance and elucidation is foolish and profitless." [14]

In the observational method, man observes what is occurring naturally; that is, nature is running the performance and controls all variables, while man is the audience. When an experiment is made, however, man assumes the part of director while retaining his role as audience, sets the stage and controls, as best he can, the pertinent variables for the purpose of testing a working hypothesis, checking a hunch, obtaining an answer to a question, or testing some general law in a definite situation. This procedure is usually spoken of as controlled experiment. In this connection, it must not be forgotten that there are degrees of control, and that it is not only more difficult to control pertinent variables, but to be aware of them, in certain sciences and in some situations than in others, for example, in biology and medicine.

After an experiment has been planned and is under way, the experimenter observes what takes place, using measures similar to those employed in the observational method. This is accomplished by means of one's unaided natural senses or through these faculties aided by the use of instruments of precision or instruments that increase the range of the natural senses, for example, electronmicroscopes and various kinds of amplifying and recording apparatus. However, in the words of Theobald Smith: "Let us not deceive ourselves concerning the true inwardness of research. It does not consist in trained senses alone. It is a quality, an attitude of the intellect working through the senses." [15] Thus, data are collected and recorded which may or may

[14] Quoted in A. L. Porterfield, *Creative Factors in Scientific Research,* Durham, N.C., 1941, p. 183.

[15] Theobald Smith, "Medical Research: Its Place in the University Medical School," *Pop. Sci. Mo.,* LXVI (1904–5), 515–30.

not be subjected to formal mathematical treatment. This is not the end, however, because an experiment must be repeated a sufficient number of times so that one may be assured that variables have been so controlled that data obtained from it approximate those of others conducted in a like manner.

At this point, it must be emphasized that one of the variables in every experiment is the experimenter, and all too frequently failure results from lack of self-control. Creative imagination in abundance is needed for formulating a problem and planning experiments for its solution, but once an experiment is under way, the investigator should switch from an imaginary realm to one of reality and with meticulous care collect and record data which then should be handled in an enthusiastically cold-blooded manner. Thus, a good scientific investigator knows when to give his imagination a loose rein, and when to bridle it thoroughly.

Not infrequently scientific methodology is "equated solely with quantitative procedures," and, if one does not use the "quantitative approach" in attempting to solve a problem, one unjustly may be considered a low-grade scientific worker. An investigator should use the procedure which seems to be most relevant to the solution of a problem without regard to whether it is quantitative or nonquantitative. According to Cantril and associates: "The establishment of any dichotomy between quantitative and nonquantitative procedure is an artificial barrier to scientific progress, separating and taking apart what really belong together in scientific method. Scientific inquiry will be strapped if the investigator feels that he cannot be scientific without being one hundred percent quantitative." [16]

After an hypothesis has been tested by experiment, the findings become a part of accumulated knowledge. But this

[16] *Science*, CX (1949), 491–97.

is not the end of scientific inquiry. The new knowledge must be integrated with the old to replace erroneous concepts, broaden those still accepted, or aid in the formation of new ones, from which new hypotheses and experiments originate. In this way, scientific inquiry is a never ending process, each step forward beginning and ending with hypotheses.

From what has been said, it might be inferred that scientific inquiry is an orderly affair always proceeding according to plan. This is far from being true. It is a fortunate scientific investigator, who, in attempting to solve a problem, quickly acquires an adequate working hypothesis. Frequently, hypotheses have to be discarded before an adequate one is formed. In addition to this, it is not always easy to find promptly a method of validating a perfectly adequate hypothesis. In such instances, the investigator plans new experiments until the proper one is devised. In case it is impossible to devise such an experiment, the investigator must wait for new discoveries or new techniques that will permit him or another worker to carry on at a later date. Poor working hypotheses and accounts of experimental failures usually do not appear in print, and those not intimately acquainted with scientific inquiry have no idea of the repeated and heartbreaking failures that precede finished products described in scientific literature.

Working hypotheses may at times lead to unexpected answers, which subsequently are substantiated. Such answers or solutions of problems should not be despised just because they were obtained by way of a poor working hypothesis. "The ability to catch hold of the wholly unforeseen and significant phenomenon is the distinctive gift of a great mind," for most of us "are mentally blind to what we do not anticipate or at least know as a possible occurrence." [17]

[17] C. S. Minot, "Certain Ideals of Medical Education," *J. Am. Med. Assn.*, LIII (1909), 502–8.

An answer to a question or a solution of a problem may be discovered by accident or it may be stumbled upon by chance. However, the value of something very precious, such as new knowledge or increased understanding, is not lessened by the fact that it was accidentally acquired. Hunches, too, play a role in scientific inquiry. The "running-back-and-forth" or the "trial-and-error" type of research also is not entirely sterile, witness some of the new, therapeutically astounding antibiotics. Although accidents, hunches, and the running-back-and-forth type of scientific research have yielded good results, even glamorous ones at times, too much emphasis should not be placed upon them.

The most important part of scientific inquiry is the investigators. What of them as a class? They are human beings and as such possess all the virtues and vices to which humanity is heir. These need not be enumerated. While there are no characteristics that set scientific investigators apart from certain other groups of workers, some occur with sufficient frequency to be mentioned. Creative imagination or originality is the most important. Disinterestedness in most things not closely related to their work is common. Many are bored by social activities, or are lonely even in the midst of acquaintances. They are highly jealous of their work in the sense that considerable effort is made to keep other activities, such as letter writing, making speeches and attending committee meetings, from interfering with it. They are meticulously honest in conducting experiments and in recording and handling data. Many work alone; others, who tolerate a few helping hands, plan and direct all activities to such an extent that the scientific growth of young men working with them is stunted; still others, with a full amount of independence, are able to surround themselves with exceptional young men and through example and provocative suggestions accelerate their development into outstanding vigorous investigators.

They are usually sensitive and modest. At times, however, I have wondered whether or not the modesty might be an affectation. Indeed, some are vain, but outspoken vanity is unusual. An investigator must firmly believe in the importance of his problem and his ability to solve it, or he will be unable to undergo the rigors and vicissitudes of scientific inquiry.

Many investigators have been accused of, or ridiculed for, retiring to ivory towers where they think and work on problems of no immediate practical importance and without due regard to what is happening in the world around them. Max Planck defended the ivory-tower worker in the following statement:

> The first step, the moulding of the world picture from its beginnings in ordinary experience, is the task of pure science. The second step, the practical utilization of the scientific world picture, is the task of technology. Both these tasks are equally important, and since either of them demands a man's full energy, if an individual scientist wants to make progress in his work, he must concentrate all his energy on one single task and for the time being forget completely other problems and interests. For this reason, never reproach the scholar too harshly for his other-worldliness and the indifference to important problems of human society. Without such a one-sided attitude, Heinrich Hertz could never have discovered radio waves, or Robert Koch the tubercle bacillus.[18]

While Planck assigned equal importance to science and the application of science, he indicated that an individual usually devotes his energy to one or the other. Nevertheless, some great investigators have evidenced competence in both. In writing of Pasteur, Dubos stated: "His life was . . . divided between the serene peace of the laboratory and the full-blooded excitement which surrounds the application of science to practical problems." [19]

[18] "The Meaning and Limits of Exact Science," *Science,* CX (1949), 319–27.
[19] *Louis Pasteur,* p. 19.

Successful scientific investigators are industrious; their working days are long, filled with toil, anxiety, and often frustration. They work hard and long because they are so eager for an answer that they cannot wait for tomorrow to continue their experiments or to begin new ones. According to Renan, a French Academician, "Nature is plebeian; she demands that one work; she prefers calloused hands and will reveal herself only to those with careworn brows." [20] To Dubos, "Science is not the product of lofty meditations and genteel behavior, it is fertilized by heartbreaking toil and long vigil—even if only too often, those who harvest the fruit are but the laborers of the eleventh hour." [21]

Hard work is an essential element of scientific inquiry. On the other hand, too much straining for solution of a problem may delay its apprehension. Some investigators think best while working with their hands, others require periods of relaxation. Helmholtz stated that happy ideas came to him unexpectedly, like an inspiration, never while at his working table, but "readily during the slow ascent of hills on a sunny day." Renan spoke beautifully of the matter in the following way:

> Truth . . . is a great coquette. She will not be won by too much passion. Indifference is often more successful with her. She escapes when apparently caught, but she yields readily if patiently waited for. She reveals herself when one is about to abandon the hope of possessing her; but she is inexorable when one affirms her, that is when one loves her with too much fervor.[22]

A scientific investigator must be an educated person. Thus, scientific inquiry has as a background not only the educated individual, but also the cultural state and educational facilities of his era and country through which he received his education. According to Welch:

[20] Quoted in *ibid.*, p. 389. [21] *Ibid.* [22] *Ibid.*

The dependence of research on education is of fundamental importance. The prime factor influencing the development of scientific research in any country is the condition of its higher education. Scientific investigation is the fruit of a tree which has its roots in the educational system, and if the roots are neglected and unhealthy, there will be no fruit. Trained investigators are bred in educational institutions.[23]

All of this means that there is a limit to the rapidity with which certain kinds of discovery can be made, and no amount of pushing or running back and forth will appreciably accelerate the process. Concepts and working hypotheses are greatly influenced by the educational and cultural state of an era in which an investigator lives. If he is sufficiently imaginative to make discoveries before society and the rest of the scientific world are prepared to accept or understand them, his findings may be disregarded or he may be proclaimed in error. Even though an investigator's concepts and hypotheses are not unduly ahead of time, he may, nevertheless, have to wait until proper techniques are devised or adequate instruments are made for testing them. Thus, when everything is ready for a discovery, it is usually made. In witness of this are the many discoveries that have been made independently and simultaneously. Of these we hear; but often we do not hear of those almost made on which work was discontinued or not reported because another investigator reached the goal first. Furthermore, it must be remembered that great discoveries are not isolated events. They are part of a chain of events consisting of the gradual accumulation of knowledge by many investigators, who may long since have died or who for other reasons are unable to be present at the forging of the last, but not necessarily the most important, link of the chain. In our enthusiasm to acclaim the hero of the hour, we often forget or

[23] W. H. Welch, "Medicine and the University," *Science,* n.s., XXVII (1908), 8–20.

fail to appreciate the careful but less spectacular work that always precedes a great discovery.

Scientific investigators as a class do not become rich. They sacrifice many of the so-called good things in life. They do not seek public acclaim, but secretly do desire the approbation of their scientific peers. Even though scientific inquiry is a very exacting spouse, most investigators have no desire to escape such tyranny. Since the path of scientific inquiry is so rugged and tedious, without obviously gainful rewards for those who use it, why do some people choose it in preference to others? Few investigators who have already died left records of the motives for making such a choice; and in most instances, living investigators, when questioned on the matter, either refuse to talk or give evasive answers. However, Cannon, during an address in 1911, made the following statement:

> The scientific investigator may not seek particularly for knowledge which can meet at once some material need. Like the artist, he is more prone to direct his efforts toward that which will for the moment properly gratify an absorbing interest of his mind. If the knowledge has, when discovered, an immediate practical value, so much the better; but the direct search for understanding has certainly always proved the most effective motive in scientific labors.[24]

If riches and public acclaim are not the usual rewards for scientific inquiry, what then is the compensation? Cannon answered the question in the following way:

> The greatest compensation, after all, for the truth seeker is the discovery of the truth. The value of labor that brings a revelation of new knowledge does not cease with the day; it remains as a permanent acquisition for the race. There is really great satisfaction to the investigator in the thought of the "durable results of the perishable years." [25]

24 W. B. Cannon, "The Career of the Investigator," *Science,* n.s., XXXIV (1911), 65–72.

25 *Ibid.*

In addition to this kind of compensation, a thrill is experienced when an investigator sees that which was imagined proved to be true. Kepler, upon completing the work that established "his third law of planetary motion," must have enjoyed the excitement and thrill which accompany scientific discovery, because he wrote convincingly concerning the matter:

What I prophesied two-and-twenty years ago, . . . what sixteen years ago I urged as a thing to be sought, . . . that for which I devoted the best part of my life to astronomical contemplations, at length I have brought to light and recognized its truth beyond my most sanguine expectations. It is not eighteen months since I got the first glimpse of light, three months since the dawn, very few days since the unveiled sun burst upon me. Nothing holds me; I will indulge my sacred fury. If you forgive, I rejoice; if you are angry, I can bear it. The die is cast, the book is written, to be read either now or by posterity, I care not which. I may well wait a century for a reader, as God has waited six thousand years for an observer.[26]

Early in this paper, I mentioned the separation of medical science from its application. At the present time, many people make a similar differentiation, but this was not the case in 1909, as evidenced by the following statement of Meltzer, one of the founders of the Harvey Society:

In years gone by, medicine was a unit and its leaders tried to master all its aspects. With the development of scientific methods and the growth of knowledge a process of differentiation took place. Heavy branches grew out of the stem of medicine, broke off and obtained an independent existence. Anatomy with all its dependencies broke away early, then followed physiology, pathologic anatomy, pharmacology and physiologic chemistry. Bacteriology tore off the branches of etiology and established itself as an independent growth. All these offsprings of medicine are now well established as pure sciences; they still closely affiliate with the mother-stem and are often designated as the sciences of medicine. What is left of the

[26] Quoted in *ibid.*

old stem is clinical medicine. What is the character of the residuum? It is generally designated as the practice of medicine. I am not aware that any one has had the courage to call it a pure science. Those who do not like to call it an art say that it is an applied science. According to this view, the relation of clinical medicine to the sciences of medicine is that of technology to science in general.[27]

At that time, Meltzer went on to make a strong plea for the extension of the process of differentiation to clinical medicine, because he was convinced that clinical medicine as it existed then was composed of two parts, one with all the elements of a pure science which should have equal rank with the other pure sciences of medicine, the other having to do with the application of science, the real practice of medicine. His plea was made in the following manner:

I entertain now and have always entertained a strong conviction that the efficiency of practise should be the supreme object in medicine. At the same time I feel sure that the efficiency of that practise will be best attained when the search for the knowledge which the practise has to use should be carried on in the same manner and by the same methods as are employed in the search for knowledge in other branches of intellectual activity. In other words, clinical research should be raised to a department of clinical science and be theoretically and practically separated to a considerable degree from the mere practical interests. . . . It will be the practise not less than the science of medicine which will benefit by such a separation.[28]

Since 1909, such a separation has been made, and Rufus Cole, by demonstrating at the Rockefeller Hospital how to accomplish it, played a very important part in bringing it about.

There are no theoretical reasons why phenomena of dis-

[27] S. J. Meltzer, "The Science of Clinical Medicine: What It Ought to Be and the Men to Uphold It," *J. Am. Med. Assn.*, LIII (1909), 508–12.
[28] *Ibid.*

ease cannot be studied scientifically in human beings. However, there are certain practical difficulties that must be overcome. Obviously, the welfare of a patient is of first importance, and his needs must be taken care of according to the best current practice of medicine. If one has too many patients and each is suffering from a different disease, one is so busy taking care of them that no time is left for scientific investigation. However, the investigator can overcome this difficulty, provided he is given an adequate salary and a suitable place to work, by undertaking at no time the care of more than a few patients. Then, since the patient is a human being and since nothing should be done to harm him, the kinds of experiment that may be conducted on him are limited. This limitation is gradually becoming less stringent because of improvements in instruments and techniques which permit a wider range of activities without harm to a patient.

For years, Cole has contended that a physician familiar with disease is the most likely person to ask of nature the best questions about disease. Consequently, he insisted that a man, before taking up clinical research seriously, should have a good medical education and at least one year, preferably two or three, of hospital experience. In addition, he urged his men to become proficient in one of the basic sciences, for example, physiology, chemistry or bacteriology, so that they themselves could apply techniques of these sciences to solution of medical problems. According to him, clinical investigators should choose problems whose most appropriate methods of attack embody techniques of which they have or can attain adequate mastery. In other words, the physician takes care of the patient and conducts the research. This does not mean that a physician may not have one or more nonmedical experts, from fields of science in which he is not adequately trained, working with him on a problem. It does mean, however, that these experts are working with and not for him, and, since he is highly trained in his own field, he has the confidence of his associates and understands why and how they attack their joint problems in certain ways. It also means that a man with clinical training alone should not hire or inveigle experts in basic sciences to do his research while he watches for reportable results.

In 1930, Cole intimated that modern medical education is turning out "an army of trained technicians," and that those who take up clinical research really do not try to learn about disease, but merely exercise their technical skill. At that time he also posed the following query: "Are they all asking questions concerning disease and attempting to solve them, or are many of them only interested in desultory and fragmentary employment of the techniques they have acquired, having faith in the Baconian concept, that if a sufficient number of observations and experiments are made, the connections will appear and general truths automatically evolve?" [29] Changes for the better have been made in the last twenty years, but too many of the faults of medical education and clinical research pointed out by Cole are still found.

For a long time to Cole and now to many others, the hospital ward is the laboratory in which clinical investigators study disease and attempt to solve medical problems, "using of course for this purpose any of the accumulated knowledge, or any technique of any science" that is suitable. This statement does not imply that activities of a clinical investigator are limited solely to hospital wards, for, according to Theobald Smith, to take a

> calm attitude toward disease as a natural phenomenon and attempt to explain it, it may be necessary to move backward

[29] *Harvey Lectures,* 1930, pp. 182–204.

toward simpler problems from man to higher animals, from these to lower types, from the complex processes of the human machine to the physical and chemical phenomena of the inorganic world. This has not always been the attitude of medicine, for standing as it does under the too near and impending shadow of suffering and death, it was but natural to attack the most difficult and complex problems first.[30]

Organized, directed research has been extolled so much recently that it cannot be disregarded. If this intense praise continues, the laity may come to believe that a discovery can be pulled by magic from a hat, or, at least, that a steering committee or research director can deliver a solution of a problem according to schedule, provided enough money, sufficient men, plenty of working space, and the latest equipment are available. Of course most people know that this is not true. Nevertheless, misconceptions about the nature of medical research are found and some take peculiar forms. For instance in 1911, according to James Ewing, a curious one "was embodied in a . . . public document recommending the introduction of the methods of the department store into scientific laboratories, as though . . . the discoveries of a Newton could be called for at a certain day and hour, or that the scientist's mind should run chiefly in the line of the card catalogue of trivial events." [31]

It must be pointed out that organized research is not a new concept, nor does it have the same meaning for different individuals. From 1651 to 1657, some of Galileo's students were banded together for investigative activities under the leadership of the Medici brothers. For ten years, 1657–1667, they constituted a large part of the well-known Accademia del Cimento, a real cooperative venture in which the members worked and published together.

[30] *Pop. Sci. Mo.*, LXVI (1904–5), 515–30.

[31] James Ewing, "The Public and the Medical Profession," *Med. Rec.*, LXXX (1911), 1209–15.

In 1905, Theobald Smith stated that "Research is in one sense a business, the laboratory a workshop. Here all sorts of processes are under way and as no one would expect a workshop to be carried on with only a foreman, so a laboratory can not be kept in use without laboratory service." By laboratory service he meant properly trained technicians. He was also aware that working space and the latest equipment are essential, but, without good investigators to use them, "are more than barren" and "create the debts rather than the assets of research." [32]

Richard Pearce, in making a plea in 1912 for organized and intensive investigation of medical problems, expressed the idea that "the individual is as important as ever" but also stated that "the laboratory . . . offers to the individual . . . advantages, facilities and opportunities, which by aiding and supplementing the work of the individual, render isolated effort unnecessary." [33] To him, organized research was exemplified by the activities in the laboratories of universities and institutes, such as the Pasteur Institute in Paris, the Institute for Infectious Diseases in Berlin, the Lister Institute for Preventive Medicine in London, the Institute for Experimental Therapeutics in Frankfort, and The Rockefeller Institute in New York City.

In 1920, James Rowland Angell wrote a paper on "The Organization of Research." [34] He was at that time chairman of the National Research Council. Moreover, World War I had been concluded about two years prior to the appearance of the article, and it is obvious that he was greatly impressed by the results obtained during the war by organized research. What he had to say then has been said repeatedly

[32] *Pop. Sci. Mo.*, LXVI (1904–5), 515–30.

[33] R. M. Pearce, "Research in Medicine, V: Medical Research in American Universities; Present Facilities, Needs and Opportunities," *Pop. Sci. Mo.*, LXXXI, 209–26.

[34] *Sci. Mo.*, XI (1920), 25–42.

by others since the end of World War II. I shall not go into details of the usual statements in favor of organized and directed research, for they must be familiar to all. Sponsors for this kind of activity are numerous and always ready to defend it. At least it seemed so to Lafayette Mendel when in 1927 he made the following remark: "Cooperative research needs no defender at the present time. It has become the cry of the hour. The preservation of individuality is the more likely to suffer neglect in a modern democracy of science." [35]

I have no particular quarrel with those in favor of organized, directed research in medicine and shall watch with interest results obtained in this manner. Up to a point, I agree with them, for the scope of research in any field has become so broad and the techniques and ways of approach to any problem are so varied that one mind cannot adequately encompass them all. Consequently, there must be some kind of organization. I would like to suggest that organization *for* research is just as effective and perhaps more so than is organized, directed research. By organization for research, I mean the provision of ample working space, good technical help, adequate facilities and equipment, proper grouping of different laboratories which are run by competent investigators with opportunities for spontaneous cooperation, and salaries for the scientific and technical workers sufficient to relieve them of personal financial worries to the extent that undivided attention can be given to problems under investigation. Laboratories of this kind should be located in universities, university medical schools and hospitals, or in institutes devoted particularly to scientific inquiry.

[35] "Some Tendencies in the Promotion of Chemical Research," *Sci.*, LXV (1927), 559–64.

In closing these remarks on organized research, I quote from Karl Deutsch's paper on "The Value of Freedom":

> Generally, the long-run promotion of abundance might require deliberate large-scale support for a *broad* development of scientific research, "pure" as well as "applied." . . . In the long run, the point may lie in the broadness of the effort rather than in its deliberate guidance in a single direction, since it is impossible to foretell in advance which new discovery not yet made will open up which new insights or new possibilities of application. Short-run compromises may have to be made in the allocation of limited scientific personnel and equipment to what appear temporarily as particularly critical tasks. But it should never be forgotten that, beyond the field of technical coordination and of gaining certain economies of scale, much of the centralized direction of scientific effort is at best a compromise with poverty, and runs the ever present risk of losing or postponing hitherto unknown new insights or discoveries of as great (or greater) importance as those which it endeavors to accelerate. Once the efficiences of coordination and large-scale efforts are given their due, it may yet appear that freedom to follow the logic of scientific theories and facts, as well as the highest abilities and interests of individuals, may have a major productive value—as well as a human value—of their own.[36]

To recapitulate, it can be said that medical research is scientific inquiry and as such should be conducted in a manner similar to that of other activities of this nature. Well-educated investigators, free to tread boldly the paths of adventure and discovery, are the most important item, but alone they can accomplish little at the present time. Well-equipped laboratories, which include research wards for clinical investigation, ample scientific and technical assistance, and an opportunity and atmosphere for cooperative effort if desirable or necessary must be at their disposal. All of this requires organization *for* but not *of*

[36] *Am. Scholar,* XVII (1948), 323–35.

research. Therefore, society must see to it that such organization is furnished so that investigators are not forced to spend a considerable part of their time arranging for it.

So much has already been accomplished through research that the "world is just now very optimistic and expectation runs high." However, the words of Theobald Smith uttered in 1905 to the effect that "If we give way to the feverish haste of our day, the slow, sure advance of medical science may be brought into discredit" [37] are more appropriate now than ever before. Moreover, haste and feverish activities may at times be mistaken for scientific results or used to cover up the fact that desired results are not being obtained.

Since this is the last of a series of papers dealing with the frontiers of medicine, one might ask: "What is the relation of medical research to these frontiers?" The medical investigator pushes the frontiers of medicine forward as he gradually clears away the jungle of unsolved problems. Thus, according to Theobald Smith: "The research worker . . . deals . . . with the undefined boundaries of knowledge and with the frayed edges of sound information. He does not march with the procession, but he must do lonely outpost and scouting duties." [38] Walter Cannon expressed the same idea in the following manner: "His chief interest is in the territory which has not yet been traversed. Indeed he is to be classed with explorers and pioneers. For such men the complacent contemplation of things accomplished is intolerable—they chafe under the routine of established ways, and find satisfactions of life in adventures beyond the frontiers." [39]

[37] *Pop. Sci. Mo.*, LXVI (1904–5), 515–30. [38] *Ibid.*

[39] "The Career of the Investigator," *Science*, n.s., XXXIV (1911), 65–72.

INDEX